A SOUND START

Solving Problems in the Teaching of Literacy

Cathy Collins Block, Series Editor

A Sound Start

Phonemic Awareness Lessons for Reading Success

CHRISTINE E. McCORMICK
REBECCA N. THRONEBURG
JEAN M. SMITLEY

THE GUILFORD PRESS
New York   London

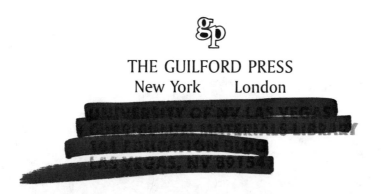

© 2002 The Guilford Press
A Division of Guilford Publications, Inc.
72 Spring Street, New York, NY 10012
www.guilford.com

Printed in the United States of America

This book is printed on acid-free paper.

Last digit is print number: 9   8   7   6   5   4   3   2   1

Library of Congress Cataloging-in-Publication Data

McCormick, Christine E.
    A sound start : phonemic awareness lessons for reading success / Christine E.
McCormick, Rebecca N. Throneberg, Jean M. Smitley.
      p. cm.—(Solving problems in the teaching of literacy)
    Includes bibliographical references (p.) and index.
    ISBN 1-57230-761-7 (pbk.)
    1. Reading—Phonetic method—United States.   2. English language—
Phonemics—Study and teaching (Early childhood)—United States.   3. Reading
(Early childhood)—United States.   I. Throneberg, Rebecca N.   II. Smitley,
Jean M.   III. Series.

LB1050.34.M33 2002
372.46′5—dc21

                                             2001055679

Illustrations by Deborah K. Reich

About the Authors

Christine E. McCormick, PhD, is a Professor in the Psychology Department at Eastern Illinois University in Charleston, where she teaches courses in developmental psychology, early childhood assessment, and early reading. She has a doctoral degree in educational psychology from the University of Minnesota and is a former Montessori teacher and school psychologist. She brings to this book over 25 years of experience in developing early reading materials for young children. Her scholarly publications include a chapter, with coauthor Jana Mason, in Teale and Sulzby's widely cited *Emergent Literacy: Reading and Writing* (Ablex, 1986). Her practical teaching resources include *Little Books, Little Books A to Z,* and *Decodable Little Books,* all published by Good Year Books, and *Fabulous Phonics Little Books,* published by Rigby.

Rebecca N. Throneburg, PhD, is an Associate Professor in the Communication Disorders and Sciences Department at Eastern Illinois University in Charleston, where she teaches courses in normal language development, phonological awareness, and language and literacy. Her doctoral degree in speech–language pathology is from the University of Illinois. She conducts research in the school setting regarding service delivery and collaboration among professionals.

Jean M. Smitley, MS, is an Associate Professor in the Communication Disorders and Sciences Department as Eastern Illinois University in Charleston, where she teaches a course in phonetics and phonological development. She has also collaborated with kindergarten teachers to provide phonological awareness training to kindergartners. Her master's degree is from Eastern Illinois University, and she has focused on reading development and disabilities in her postgraduate course work.

Preface

Developing awareness of the sounds of spoken language—skills of phonemic awareness—is now known to enhance learning to read and to be an important part of the early reading curriculum (National Reading Panel, 2000). This book provides lessons and materials for teaching the skills of phonemic awareness. The lessons are intended to be used as one component of a broad early reading program.

Three packages of lessons are provided. The first set of phonemic awareness lessons was developed for the whole class and small groups. The second set of phonemic awareness lessons was developed for those few children who need additional, more intensive instruction because of minimal progress with class and small-group lessons. The third set provides class lessons on the auditory, visual, and motoric properties of English consonant phonemes. Each set of lessons includes specific directions and materials. Assessment measures are provided for each of the first two sets of lessons. The organized, structured lessons should be especially helpful for teachers beginning to add instruction in phonemic awareness skills to their early reading program.

The goal of the lessons is to help all children develop the phonemic awareness skills that promote success with learning to read. Children's varying responses to instruction can be accommodated. In Chapter 3 the small-group lessons, each of which accompanies a whole-class lesson, provide additional practice on the same skills taught in the whole-class lesson and may be used with the entire class or only with those children needing additional practice. The set of individualized lessons in Chapter 5 can then provide more intensive instruction for children with difficulties in developing awareness of phonemes, the individual sounds within words. In Chapter 6 the set of whole-class lessons on the production of phonemes can supplement instruction on awareness of phonemes and letter sounds.

All sets of lessons were used successfully and enjoyably by the authors and other teachers for more than 3 years. While the lessons were developed with kindergarten children, the appropriate age range is wider than kindergarten (see the accompanying table on applicability of lessons by grade level). In Chapter 3 the first 10 of the whole-class and small-group lessons, which emphasize skills of rhyming and syllable awareness, are also appropriate for prekindergarten children; the second 10 of the whole-class and small-group lessons on phoneme level skills are also appropriate for nonreading first-grade children. In Chapter 5 the individualized lessons for children showing special difficulty with awareness of phonemes can be used with second-semester kindergarten children or nonreading first-grade children.

In Chapter 1 we present an overview of phonemic awareness including a description of its nature, how phonemic awareness skills are related to learning to read, its usual developmental sequence, assessment and general instructional issues, and why some children need individualized, more intensive instruction.

Chapter 2, which introduces the whole-class and small-group lessons, includes guidelines for the lessons, a description of the developmental sequence of skills in the lessons, the plan of the lessons, and the assessment measure to be used with the lessons. The lessons are set up for a weekly whole-class lesson and small-group or center activities, but this format can be modified depending on your curriculum and personnel resources, as well as your comfort with embedding the skills in whole-class activities.

Chapter 3 provides the 20 sequential lessons to be presented across the kindergarten year. (As already noted, the first 10 lessons are appropriate for prekindergarten children, and the last 10 are also appropriate for nonreading first-grade children.) Each lesson is introduced using a familiar children's book and integrates a variety of activities and materials for the skills of that lesson. Small-group activities for the same skills accompany each lesson. Additional related activities are also suggested for embedding the skills in other whole-class activities. Although the lessons are primarily auditory in nature, print is included throughout to emphasize the link of phonemic awareness skills to preparation for learning to read. All needed materials are included with each lesson except for the storybooks and nonreproducible materials for the activities.

Chapter 4 begins with a review of the need for an additional level of instruction for those children showing minimal progress in the whole-class and small-group lessons on skills of awareness of phonemes. The skills taught in this second set of individualized lessons are awareness of specific phonemes and their match to letters. Directions for identifying children needing this additional instruction, an overview of the sequence of lessons, and an assessment measure to be used with these lessons are included.

Chapter 5 presents the 16 individualized lessons, about 15 minutes each, which can readily be used with individual children or groups of two or three children. Scripted directions are provided, and all needed materials accompany each lesson. In these lessons the children are highly interactive with the teacher, and the lessons allow for close monitoring of each child's progress.

Applicability of Lessons by Grade Level

Grade	Whole-class and small group (Chapter 3)	Individualized (Chapter 5)	Phoneme characteristics (Chapter 6)
Prekindergarten	First or second semester: Lessons 1–10		First and second semesters: Phoneme lessons /b/ to /z/—information for children and listening for sound by itself
Kindergarten	First semester: Lessons 1–10; second semester: Lessons 11–20	Second semester: Lessons 1–16	First and second semesters: All lessons (in teacher's sequence of letter-sound introduction)
First grade	First semester: Lessons 11–20	First or second semester (with nonreaders): Lessons 1–16	First and second semesters: All lessons as phonemes and corresponding letters are reviewed

Chapter 6 begins with general information for the teacher about the phonemes in English, such as how each phoneme is produced in the mouth. Each of the 22 phoneme lessons can be presented to give the class additional information about the acoustic features and production of phonemes during your usual alphabetic letter-sound instruction. Helping children to become familiar with the place and manner of the phonemes' articulation can assist them in learning and anchoring the phonemes' identities.

This resource book provides an organized and systematic approach to teaching phonemic awareness skills. Each of the three sets of lessons can be used independently or in coordination with each other. We have attempted to provide a resource that allows teachers to readily begin including phonemic awareness in their early reading program by providing directions and materials for each lesson. We have found the lessons to be effective, engaging, and fun for children, and we hope that this book will allow you and your students to have the same enjoyable and fruitful learning experience.

REFERENCE

National Reading Panel. (2000). *Report of the National Reading Panel: Reports of the subgroups.* Washington, DC: National Institute of Child Health and Human Development Clearinghouse. NIH Pub. No. 00-4754.

Acknowledgments

We wish to thank the kindergarten teachers and speech pathologists of the Charleston, Illinois, Community Unit 1 School District for their help over the years as we developed the lessons in this book. Special thanks to Millie Fleming and Cheryl Todd and their students for working with us so enthusiastically. We also wish to thank the graduate students in the Communication Disorders and Sciences Department and the Psychology Department at Eastern Illinois University for their help in developing the lessons. Many thanks to Deb Reich, Pam Gutowski, and Sarah Weaver for their assistance in preparing the manuscript.

Contents

A SOUND START

Chapter 1

Phonemic Awareness: An Introduction

A primary consensus from the last 20 years of research on learning to read is that skills of phonemic awareness, or skills in attending to the sounds of speech, are highly predictive of learning to read. The National Reading Panel's meta-analysis of the experimental research on phonemic awareness confirms that teaching skills of phonemic awareness increases subsequent reading achievement (Ehri et al., 2001). Phonemes, the separable sounds within words, are the smallest unit of phonemic awareness skill and the unit most directly related to success with learning to read (Hoien, Lundberg, Stanovich, & Bjaalid, 1995; Share, Jorm, Maclean, & Matthews, 1984).

Note that the term "phonemic awareness" is often used interchangeably with the term "phonological awareness" (International Reading Association, 1998). To be more exact, phonological awareness is the more general term and refers to all units of sounds in speech from the larger units such as the word and syllable to the smallest unit of individual sounds, the phonemes. When both terms are used, phonemic awareness is the more specific term for awareness of phonemes only. We use the term phonemic awareness in this book to encompass all units of sound in speech because the term is frequently used in this manner in the literature and in discussions of these skills, such as in the introduction to the curriculum by Adams, Foorman, Lundberg, and Beeler (1998).

Children who readily learn to read have acquired skills of phonemic awareness, although these skills were often not recognized or labeled as phonemic awareness. To illustrate the nature of these skills as they may develop in children with rich early language experiences, consider the following example: At age 4, the son of one of the authors would often include rhyming words in his everyday talk. For instance, one day when his mom suggested they go shopping, he replied, "What? Go shopping, wopping, bopping, Mom?" In addition to verbal play with rhyming words, many young children also love the alliteration and rhyme in books, such as Dr. Seuss books and many alphabet books. This delight in the sounds of words reflects emerging skills in phonemic awareness. Children showing these behaviors are beginning to attend to the sound structure of language rather than the meaning of speech as we do in usual conversation.

At a more sophisticated level of phonemic awareness skill, consider Ashley, a 4½-year-old. While playing at the home of one of the authors a number of years ago, she was sitting with a magnetic alphabet and putting the letters into their frame. As Ashley placed the *Q* in sequence she said, "You know, I have a *Q* in my name. *Q*, Candace. Ashley Candace, *Q* for Candace." She clearly demonstrated emerging skill in what now is termed awareness of phonemes. She knew that words (her middle name, in this example) began with a specific sound. Plus, she was beginning to match that awareness of beginning sounds in words to a specific letter. (Although *Q* was not the correct letter, Ashley's choice was phonemically accurate. That is, the letter *Q* has a /k/ sound in it, as does Candace.) She was on her way, even before kindergarten, to understanding how our alphabet works to represent the sounds of language. These examples of children's interest in the sounds of language demonstrate that, although the term phonemic awareness is fairly recent, the skills have been present all along in young children when they have early language environments which include plenty of shared book reading and verbal play with the sounds in words (Snow, Burns, & Griffin, 1998).

The empirical evidence for the causal influence of these oral language skills on learning to read is clear (Ehri et al., 2001). Instruction which helps children attend to the sounds of spoken words (that the speech stream can be separated into words, syllables, beginning sounds, rhymes, and individual sounds) enhances learning to read for all children and is especially important for children who are not informally developing these skills and require explicit instruction to do so (Torgesen & Mathes, 2000).

PHONEMIC AWARENESS AND LEARNING TO READ

The goal of teaching phonemic awareness skills is to better prepare children for success with learning to read and thus help to prevent early reading failure (Ehri at al., 2001; Snow et al., 1998). Learning to accurately identify or decode printed words is a primary task for the beginning reader (Gough, 1996). Effective phonemic awareness instruction and teaching the matches between a phoneme and a letter facilitate decoding abilities in beginning readers by helping children understand the way words in oral language are represented in print (Torgesen & Mathes, 2000).

Understanding how spoken words are represented in print requires at least three skills: (1) Children need to know that words are made of separable sounds (awareness of phonemes). (2) They need to know the letters of our alphabet well. (3) They need to understand the specific matches between sounds and letters in words. Understanding that specific letters represent specific sounds is called the alphabetic principle and allows the beginning reader to develop the useful decoding strategy of "sounding out" printed words to identify them. A lack of understanding this principle may explain why about 25% of mid-first grade children do not catch on to phonics instruction, which teaches the systematic relationships between letters and their sounds (Adams, Treiman, & Pressley, 1998).

While letter name knowledge is also essential for learning the alphabetic principle, learning the letter names is a more straightforward task. With sufficient instruction and practice, including time for children to experiment with writing letters for sounds in words, children can learn them. However, some children memorize letter names and their corresponding sounds without the awareness that spoken words are composed of separable sounds. These are the children likely to encounter problems with learning to "sound out" and blend individual letter sounds into words because they have difficulty separating words into phonemes (Adams, Treiman, et al., 1998).

INSTRUCTION IN PHONEMIC AWARENESS

Curricular materials for explicit instruction in phonemic awareness generally follow the developmental sequence of young children's emerging skills in phonemic awareness. This sequence of development usually proceeds from the larger and easier-to-recognize units of words and syllables to the smaller and more difficult-to-hear unit of the phoneme. Thus, instruction begins with activities developing awareness of words, rhymes, and syllables, and then proceeds to initial and final sounds in words and finally all phonemes within words. As well, in order to provide the greatest positive effect on learning to read, the match between specific letters and phonemes is essential (Ehri et al., 2001). Because in preschool and at the start of kindergarten most children are not yet readers, nearly all children can benefit from increasing these skills through appropriate instructional activities which are engaging and fun (Snow et al., 1998; Torgesen & Mathes, 2000).

Curricular suggestions and materials for teaching phonemic awareness skills are increasingly available, as the following examples illustrate: Yopp (1995a) provides an annotated bibliography for books that deal playfully with speech sounds. A wide variety of informal activities which play with sounds in words through songs, chants, and games are described by Yopp (1992) and Yopp and Yopp (2000). These authors suggest that the teacher embed such informal play activities in meaningful language instruction throughout the day, and they recommend explicitly connecting phonemes with letters. Encouraging invented or temporary spelling, by which children use the sounds in words to spell, has been shown to be an effective method of teaching awareness of phonemes (Scanlon & Vellutino, 1997). Ericson and Juliebo's (1998) description of activities for embedding phonemic awareness instruction includes a general plan for activities over the course of the kindergarten year and specific suggestions for beginning the connection between letters and phonemes. Adams, Foorman, et al. (1998) provide a large set of more structured activities with an extensive research base in their phonemic awareness curriculum.

The aforementioned materials require the teacher to select activities to incorporate into instruction. Teachers less comfortable with selecting and embedding phonemic awareness into class activities may find the sequential, scripted phonemic awareness lessons in this book especially helpful. As well, reproducible materials accompany each lesson.

Children vary widely in their response to instruction (Torgesen & Mathes, 2000; Yopp, 1992, 1995b). Some will readily acquire phonemic awareness skills in class lessons, and others will struggle with developing these skills.

Child variability is of special importance regarding awareness of phonemes, because identifying phonemes is difficult for many children. One reason is that phonemes are not easily separable in the speech stream and often blend with the surrounding phonemes. (In contrast, syllables are much easier to identify than phonemes because syllables are punctuated in the speech stream and thus provide an obvious cue.) Identifying phonemes can be especially troublesome to children with limited general language skills and difficulties in processing the sounds of language—that is, phonological processing (Adams, Treiman, et al., 1998; Torgesen, 2000).

Difficulties in phonological processing may be reflected by minimal progress with class phonemic awareness instruction and slowness or lack of fluency in learning letter names and letter sounds. Provision of class instruction and monitoring the children's progress can help to identify those children lacking exposure to activities which stimulate phonemic awareness (and likely to respond well to class and small-group instruction), distinguishing such children from those with impaired phonological processing abilities (and likely to need additional, intensive instruction). With explicit whole-class teaching of phonemic awareness skills and additional supportive instruction for those children showing minimal progress with class instruction, early reading problems can be reduced (Snow et al., 1998).

ASSESSMENT OF PHONEMIC AWARENESS

Assessment of phonemic awareness skills can be approached in several ways (Torgesen & Mathes, 2000). Standardized norm-referenced measures compare a child's performance to that of a larger representative group of children the same age. Scores from a standardized test give the teacher information about the general level of development in the class, as well as the skills of individual children. Examples of standardized tests include the individually administered *Phonological Awareness Test* (Robertson & Salter, 1997), with multiple measures of awareness of phonemes, and the shorter small-group-administered *Test of Phonological Awareness* (TOPA) (Torgesen & Bryant, 1994). Informal measures assess which skills the child can perform; the Yopp–Singer Test of Phoneme Segmentation (Yopp, 1995b) is one example. Informal tests are especially useful for monitoring children's progress with a specific curriculum (Torgesen & Mathes, 2000). The assessment measures developed to accompany both the class and individualized lessons in this resource book are examples of informal measures that can be used to monitor the children's progress with the lessons.

For a more in-depth discussion of phonemic awareness assessment issues and recommended measures, see Torgesen and Mathes (2000). Additionally, *A Practical Guide to Reading Assessments* (International Reading Association, 2000) describes a broader range of assessment measures but does not discuss general measurement issues as do Torgesen and Mathes (2000).

At the beginning of the kindergarten year, some children in the class may be proficient in phonemic awareness skills of rhyming or even awareness of phonemes at the beginning of words. Other children may have no skills in noticing the sounds of spoken words. Using the assessment measure accompanying the class lessons in Chapter 2 (before beginning instruction) gives the teacher information about the variability of skills within the class, information that is useful for adapting instruction to the needs of the class. For example, if most of the children demonstrate little or no phonemic awareness skill, that will indicate a need for emphasis on the developmentally early skills of rhyme and syllable awareness; if the majority of the class is proficient in these skills, then they can be progressed through quickly—with more instruction given only to those children with minimal skills.

Assessment at the beginning of the second semester of kindergarten can identify the children who are showing minimal progress with class instruction and who need additional, more intensive instruction. After a semester of instruction, as long as the phoneme level of lessons has begun, it is the children with limited general-language development and/or specific difficulties with phonological processing who are most likely to be experiencing difficulty with awareness of phonemes.

At the end of the kindergarten year, assessment can be used to measure the progress of the class and individual children to determine the effectiveness of the lessons. It can also identify those children likely to need additional support in first grade during systematic reading instruction.

GENERAL INSTRUCTIONAL ISSUES

1. It is important to explicitly include phonemic awareness instruction as a regular part of curriculum. Letter instruction should also be included because letter knowledge is essential for transfer of phonemic awareness skills to reading and spelling. At the same time, phonemic awareness instruction ought to be only one part of a much broader early reading program which should include shared book reading, language enrichment and vocabulary activities, and time for play and experimentation with the letters and their sounds (Adams, Treiman, et al., 1998; Ehri et al., 2001; Torgesen & Mathes, 2000).

2. While lessons in phonemic awareness are often similar to activities in which many teachers engage with young children, the conscious and explicit attention to the phonological or sound structure of oral language is necessary for at least 25% of children to acquire these skills (Torgesen &

Mathes, 2000). This instruction should be presented through fun and engaging activities as an enjoyable component of the early reading curriculum and should accommodate the instructional needs of the class (Snow et al., 1998; Torgesen & Mathes, 2000).

3. Lessons need to begin with the earlier levels of phonemic awareness, proceed to the phoneme level, and include the match of phonemes to letters. The earlier levels of phonemic awareness, such as rhyme and syllable awareness, usually develop before the phoneme level; yet rhyme and syllable skills are less directly related to learning to read than awareness of phonemes (Hoien et al., 1995).

4. Absolute levels of these skills needed for success with learning to read are not well established. This is an ongoing research question, and we know that, while phonemic awareness instruction enhances reading acquisition, it continues to develop during the first year of reading instruction; there is a reciprocal relationship (Adams, Treiman, et al., 1998). As a guideline, Torgesen and Mathes (2000) suggest that, by the end of kindergarten, awareness of beginning sounds in words and blending two and three phonemes into words appear to reflect adequate phonemic awareness skills for systematic instruction in beginning reading.

5. A few children will need additional support beyond class instruction. Phonemes are especially difficult for children with limited phonological processing skills. Providing more intensive instruction (in addition to whole-class and small-group instruction) on phonemes can increase these children's likelihood of success with learning to decode. At the same time, even with this additional instruction, a small percentage of children will continue to require intensive instruction as they learn to read (Torgesen, 2000).

6. The phonemes of the English language need to be pronounced correctly when modeled to children. This may sound easy but is actually quite challenging with some sounds. Distortions or errors in phoneme production can affect children's ability to perceive and blend sounds. One of the most common errors when pronouncing the consonant sounds is to add a vowel (usually the sound /uh/, called the schwa vowel) after the sounds. Adding the vowel makes the sound seem louder so that children will hear it. For example, the sound that the letter *s* makes is a long continuous stream of air: /sssss/. Because it is a quiet, voiceless sound, some people mistakenly pronounce the sound the *s* makes as /sssss*uh*/. Teaching phonemic awareness requires a good understanding of the phonemes of our language.

THE LESSONS IN THIS BOOK

This resource book provides three sets of easy-to-implement lessons with scripted directions and reproducible materials accompanying each lesson. All sets of lessons have been taught effectively by the authors, classroom teachers, and speech–language therapists for 3 years and are consistent with the instructional approaches described by the National Reading Panel (2000). The scripted lessons are especially helpful for teachers just beginning to explicitly teach phonemic awareness skills. With experience, teachers may find less need to follow the scripts and become more adept at creating their own activities to meet the particular needs of the children in their class.

Each sequential class lesson in Chapter 3 includes an approximately 30-minute introduction and activity for the entire class and a small-group lesson on the same skill. The class lessons begin with awareness of words, rhymes, and syllables in Lessons 1–10, and proceed to the phonemes in Lessons 11–20. Depending on the needs of the class, the small-group activity can be used with all children or only those children needing the additional practice with the skill introduced in the class lesson. An assessment measure developed to monitor children's progress is included in the introduction to the class lessons in Chapter 2.

The individualized lessons in Chapter 5 can be used in the second semester of kindergarten (or beginning first grade) with those few children who are showing minimal progress on awareness of initial phonemes in words in class instruction. The 16 sequential lessons, of about 15 minutes each, focus on a small set of phonemes and their matching letters. The lessons can be used with individual children or groups of two or three children by a classroom teacher, reading teacher, or speech–language pathologist. (Often the children needing this level of instruction are also receiving speech services.) An assessment measure developed to accompany these lessons is included in the introduction to the lessons in Chapter 4.

Chapter 6 begins with general information for the teacher about the place, manner, and voicing articulatory characteristics of consonant phonemes in English. With more in-depth knowledge of phonemic awareness, such as explicit discussion of how particular phonemes are made by the mouth, children are better able to understand the similarities and differences among the phonemes. Tips for the pronunciation of sounds and scripted class lessons for describing and identifying 22 consonant phonemes are presented.

The chapters that follow include guidelines, lessons, and materials to help you provide effective instruction for all children.

REFERENCES

Adams, M., Foorman, B., Lundberg, I., & Beeler, C. (1998). *Phonemic awareness in young children: A classroom curriculum*. Baltimore: Brookes.

Adams, M., Treiman, R., & Pressley, M. (1998). Reading, writing and literacy. In I. Sigel & K. Renninger (Eds.), *Handbook of child psychology* (5th ed., pp. 275–355). New York: Wiley.

Ehri, L. C., Nunes, S. R., Willows, D. M., Schuster, B. B., Yaghoub-Zadeh, Z., & Shanahan, T. (2001). Phonemic awareness instruction helps children learn to read: Evidence from the National Reading Panel's meta-analysis. *Reading Research Quarterly, 36*(3), 250–283.

Ericson, L., & Juliebo, M. F. (1998). *Phonological awareness handbook for kindergarten and primary grade teachers*. Newark, DE: International Reading Association.

Gough, P. B. (1996). How children learn to read and why they fail. *Annals of Dyslexia, 46*, 3–20.

Hoien, T., Lundberg, I., Stanovich, K. E., & Bjaalid, I. (1995). Components of phonological awareness. *Reading and Writing: An Interdisciplinary Journal, 7*, 171–188.

International Reading Association. (1998). *Phonemic awareness and learning to read* [Position Statement]. Newark, DE: Author.

International Reading Association. (2000). *A practical guide to reading assessments*. Newark, DE: Author.

National Reading Panel. (2000). *Report of the National Reading Panel: Reports of the subgroups*. Washington, DC: National Institute of Child Health and Human Development Clearinghouse.

Robertson, C., & Salter, W. (1997). *The Phonological Awareness Test*. East Moline, IL: LinguiSystems.

Scanlon, D. M., & Vellutino, F. R. (1997). A comparison of the instructional backgrounds and cognitive profiles of poor, average, and good readers who were initially identified as at risk for reading failure. *Scientific Studies of Reading, 1*, 191–216.

Share, D., Jorm, A., Maclean, R., & Matthews, R. (1984). Sources of individual differences in reading acquisition. *Journal of Educational Psychology, 76*, 1309–1324.

Snow, C. E., Burns, M. S., & Griffin, P. (Eds.). (1998). *Preventing reading difficulties in young children*. Washington, DC: National Academy Press.

Torgesen, J. K. (2000). Individual differences in response to early interventions in reading: The lingering problem of treatment resisters. *Learning Disabilities Research and Practice, 15*(1), 55–64.

Torgesen, J. K., & Bryant, B. (1994). *Test of Phonological Awareness*. Austin, TX: PRO-ED.

Torgesen, J. K., & Mathes, P. G. (2000). *A basic guide to understanding, assessing and teaching phonological awareness*. Austin, TX: PRO-ED.

Yopp, H. K. (1992). Developing phonemic awareness in young children. *The Reading Teacher, 45*(9), 696–703.

Yopp, H. K. (1995a). Read-aloud books for developing phonemic awareness: An annotated bibliography. *The Reading Teacher, 48*(6), 538–543.

Yopp, H. K. (1995b). A test for assessing phonemic awareness in young children. *The Reading Teacher, 49*(1), 20–29.

Yopp, H. K., & Yopp, R. H. (2000). Supporting phonemic awareness development in the classroom. *The Reading Teacher, 54*(2), 130–143.

Chapter 2

Introduction to the Whole-Class
and Small-Group Lessons

GENERAL GUIDELINES

Chapter 3 contains whole-class and small-group lessons for instruction of phonemic awareness skills that can be used by preschool, kindergarten, or first-grade teachers. These lessons should be taught as one part of a broader early reading curriculum. Although the classroom teacher may independently deliver the phonemic awareness lessons, collaboration with other professionals such as speech–language pathologists, reading resource teachers, or school psychologists might also be considered. Many professionals are aware of the critical link between phonemic awareness skills success and learning to read. These professionals can assist with delivery of the small-group component of these lessons or might well be helpful in brainstorming modifications that can be made to the large-group lessons to fit the needs of your class.

Children need to develop a working knowledge as well as a conscious understanding of the sounds and sound structure of our language. Explicitly explaining the vocabulary and concepts related to the various phonological awareness tasks (e.g., blending, syllables, rhyme) is important. At a workshop recently, an audience member asked if we used the word "syllable" in a kindergarten class or if we just referred to syllables as parts of words. It was explained that it is necessary to use the terms (e.g., syllable, word, rhyme, sound, letter) to define the target area along with a definition the children can understand (e.g., the parts of a word). A kindergarten teacher with whom one of the authors collaborates reported a child asking his mother in the car, "Mom, do you know how many syllables are in the word hippopotamus?" This example shows that the child is beginning to understand how to think about words independent of their meaning.

SEQUENCE OF SKILLS

The following lessons are based on developmental information (Moats, 2000) and the authors' own experiences in presenting these lessons. It takes varying time and practice for children to develop the ability to attend to the sounds in a word and to manipulate these sounds.

We have designed the 20 whole-class lessons so that the first 10 focus on the larger unit phonemic awareness skills (e.g., rhyming, word/syllable awareness, onset–rime) and Lessons 11–20 focus on the phoneme (e.g., isolation of beginning, middle and ending sounds; phoneme counting, blending, and segmenting).

An outline of the skills targeted each week is listed below:

Week	Area targeted
1	Concept of words
2	Rhyme recognition and discrimination
3	Rhyme choice
4	Rhyme production
5	Syllable awareness/counting
6	Syllable blending
7	Syllable deletion
8	Onset–rime blending
9	Onset–rime blending
10	Review/assessment of rhyme production, blending syllables, and blending onset–rime
11	Initial sound identification
12	Initial sound production
13	Final sound identification
14	Final sound production
15	Medial sound production
16	Phoneme counting
17	Phoneme blending
18	Phoneme blending
19	Phoneme segmentation
20	Review/assessment of initial, medial, and final sound identification; phoneme counting, segmenting, blending, and deleting

The teacher should feel free to adapt the activities in each lesson to the class response. For example, if many children in the class are experiencing difficulty blending onsets and rimes into words, the teacher may wish to spend one more week on that skill. Also, suggestions for additional related activities are provided for each lesson so that the teacher can provide more practice on any skill necessary to meet the needs of the class.

PLAN OF THE LESSONS

The whole-class lessons presented here should take approximately 30 minutes. Beginning with an introduction to the specific skill, the teacher should explicitly state and explain the skill. The introduction to the various phonemic awareness skills is necessary to describe the task to the class. The introduction is the time when children are focused and presentation of multiple examples of the skill can be given. For example, we have had three people be a train (engine, train car, and caboose) and chug in front of the classroom. First, the engine says a sound, next the train car says a sound, and then the caboose says a sound; finally the class blends the phonemes into a word. Materials such as puppets and objects are suggested to make the introduction informative yet enjoyable.

We have included literature with these lessons to help link phonemic awareness to reading. The stories allow children to look at pictures, follow a sequence of events, listen to oral speech, and practice phonemic awareness skills. The literature also often provides a theme which is then incorporated in whole-class or small-group activities. The books included in these lessons are available in most libraries. Alternative books and a listing of the materials needed for each lesson are included in the Appendix.

The whole-class activities provide a simple way to ensure that all children have the opportunity to develop these phonemic awareness skills. The children are often active during these activities and take turns manipulating words, sounds, etc. Sometimes the children participate by responding to or vocalizing particular sounds, words, or syllables during activities. Music, gross motor activity (e.g., jumping or clapping to syllables), and visual stimuli help the children realize that it can be fun to analyze words. It is suggested that children sit in circles for some of the whole-class activities, but that may not be possible dependent upon the size of the classroom. Be flexible in adapting the lesson to fit the needs of the children in the class.

The small-group activity can be used for all children in the class if you have enough time to implement multiple small groups throughout the week. An alternative is to invite assistants (parents, teacher assistants, speech pathologists, or other professionals) to help, with each adult instructing a small group simultaneously. You may also decide that your time and resources allow for only one or two small-group lessons. The small-group lessons can then be used to provide extra assistance to the children in your class who seem to be struggling with the concepts presented in the whole-class format. Use the assessment data along with classroom performance to determine which small group or groups of children are most in need of additional practice.

DATA ON EFFECTIVENESS

Phonemic awareness lessons equivalent to the ones included in this book were provided in two kindergarten classrooms during the 1997/98 school year. In the first classroom, all children received the whole-class and small-group components of the phonemic awareness lessons. The lessons were collaboratively taught by the classroom teacher, a speech–language pathologist, and other teaching assistants. In the second classroom, the classroom teacher independently presented the whole-class lessons and other related activities, but none of the children received small-group instruction. In both of the first two classrooms where phonemic awareness was taught, the classroom teacher also taught a letter-sound/letter-name approach to early reading instruction. In a third classroom, the classroom teacher provided a letter-sound/letter-name approach to early reading instruction without a phonemic awareness component. All of the children in the three classes were tested at the beginning and end of kindergarten with the *Phonological Awareness Test* (PAT) (Robertson & Salter, 1997). The mean gain of the class that received both the whole-class and small-group lessons was 50 points. The mean gain of the class that received only the whole-class lessons and related activities was 33 points. The mean gain of the class that received the traditional instruction without a phonemic awareness component was 14 points (Barnes, Smitley, & Throneburg, 1998).

During the 1999/2000 school year the whole-class and small-group lessons were provided in four kindergarten classrooms. All children were individually assessed with the *Phonological Aware-*

ness Literacy Screening (PALS) with the exceptions of the individual rhyme and concept of word sections (Invernizzi & Meier, 1997). The test evaluated skills of rhyming, initial sound identification, letter-sound knowledge, and single-word reading and spelling. Figure 2.1 presents each of the four classrooms' test scores at the beginning and end of the year as well as the difference or gain between the two tests. On the total test score, 112 points were possible. More than 80 children participated in the lessons from the four classes. At the end of the year, most of the children in these classes evidenced substantial gains in the skills during kindergarten, with average class posttest scores that were more than four times greater than average pretest scores. Only six children (7%) were significantly below the class means at the end of the school year (Throneburg, Smitley, & Hilgenberg, 2000).

ASSESSMENT

Assessment of phonemic awareness skills can be accomplished through a number of published assessment tools, such as the PAT, or by informal means. It is recommended that the assessment include evaluation of rhyming, syllable and phoneme blending, as well as initial and final sound identification.

We have included a brief 26-item informal assessment of these phonemic awareness skills at the end of this chapter: 8 items evaluate rhyming judgment and production; 10 items evaluate blending syllables, onset–rime, and phonemes; and 8 items evaluate initial and final sound identification. This assessment also contains three optional sections that evaluate phonics/sound–letter knowledge. The optional section includes 19 items to evaluate sound–letter skills, 5 items to evaluate the ability to read words that can be phonetically decoded, and 5 items to evaluate writing single words that can be phonetically segmented. Two sets of all the test items are included. One set can be used as a pretest of skills, and a second set can be used later as a posttest of skills to evaluate skill growth over the school year.

The phonemic awareness assessment should be administered individually to children. The

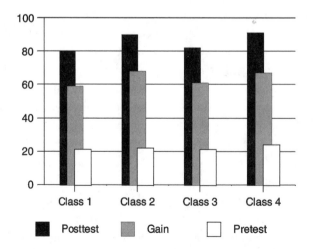

FIGURE 2.1. Average class scores on the Phonological Awareness Literacy Screening (PALS) before and after class lessons.

nonoptional sections (rhyming, blending, and phoneme identification) usually require less than 10 minutes per child. The average time for the optional sound–letter, reading, and writing sections also varies with the skill of the child, but most children complete the tasks in 5–10 minutes. The optional section is strongly recommended by the end of kindergarten. The assessment may be administered by a teacher, teacher aide, speech–language pathologist, or other education professional. The professional who administers the assessment should be aware of the proper production of speech sounds. (Say individual phonemes without adding a schwa vowel—e.g., /sss/ like a snake sound, not /suh/; /f/, just air blowing, not /fuh/.) Detailed information about the phonemes in the English/American language and the correct pronunciation of the sounds is included in Chapter 6.

REFERENCES

Barnes, C., Smitley, J. [M.], & Throneburg, R. [N.] (1998). *Phonological awareness training: Effects on phonological awareness and reading skills.* Paper presented at the National Convention of the American Speech–Language–Hearing Association.

Invernizzi, M., & Meier, J. (1997). *Phonological Awareness Literacy Screening.* Charlottesville: University of Virginia Press.

Moats, L. C. (2000). *Speech to print.* Baltimore: Brookes.

Robertson, C., & Salter, W. (1997). *The Phonological Awareness Test.* East Moline, IL: LinguiSystems.

Throneburg, R. N., Smitley, J. S., & Hilgenberg, K. (2000). *Individual student differences in phonological awareness training in kindergarten.* Paper presented at the National Convention of the American Speech–Language–Hearing Association.

Phonemic Awareness Assessment

Child's name _____   Pretest date _____

Teacher's name _____   Posttest date _____

There is a line following each item on the test. The examiner may indicate with a +/– the correctness of the response or may record the child's actual response on the line.

RHYMING

Instructions/Practice

The first thing we are going to do is work with some rhyming words. Words rhyme when the ends of the words sound the same. For example, "pot" and "hot" rhyme. "Pot" and "hot" both have the sounds "ot" at the end of the words. Now listen to these words "bag," "rake"—they don't rhyme because they sound different at the ends of the words (*pause between initial sound and rest of word*) "b–ag," "r–ake." Let's think of a word that rhymes with "cat" (*let the child respond and give him or her feedback as to why response was correct or incorrect*). Now I am going to ask you about some more rhyming words, but I won't be able to help you. Don't worry if you don't know all the answers; go ahead and take your best guess about each answer.

Rhyming Judgment

Listen to these words and tell me if the two words rhyme or don't rhyme with each other.

Pretest	*Posttest*
1. lake–cake	1. pig–dig
2. cat–dog	2. hop–sad
3. red–bed	3. mat–sat
4. fox–box	4. five–pink

Rhyming Production

Next I'm going to say a word, and I want you to think of a word that rhymes with it. The word you think of can be a real word or a silly made-up word. For example, if I say the word "show," words that you can say that rhyme with it are "toe, mow, go, coe, low, doe, poe." You only need to tell me one word that rhymes with the word I say. Tell me a word that rhymes with . . .

5. pop	_____	5. shoe	_____
6. sun	_____	6. win	_____
7. light	_____	7. mat	_____
8. rice	_____	8. bake	_____

Total correct
rhyme pretest ___/8_

Total correct
rhyme posttest ___/8_

BLENDING

Instructions/Examples

Next I'm going to say some pieces of words, and you need to listen very carefully and put the pieces together to figure out the secret words I'm saying. For example, if I say (*pause ½–1 second between segments*) "gi–raffe," you can put the pieces together and tell me the secret word is "giraffe." If I say "d–og," you can tell me the secret word I said was "dog."

Syllables

Pretest		*Posttest*	
1. play-ground	_____	1. base-ball	_____
2. bas-ket	_____	2. ta-ble	_____
3. am-bu-lance	_____	3. hel-i-cop-ter	_____

Onset–Rime

(*Say individual phonemes without adding schwa vowel—i.e., /sss/ like a snake sound, not /suh/; f, just air blowing, not /fuh/.*)

4. f-all	_____	4. p-ot	_____
5. b-ake	_____	5. s-and	_____
6. s-un	_____	6. c-oat	_____
7. c-at	_____	7. f-ish	_____

Phonemes

8. p-i-g	_____	8. b-oa-t	_____
9. c-a-n	_____	9. k-i-te	_____
10. f-i-ght	_____	10. s-i-t	_____

Total correct
   blending pretest ___/10

Total correct
   blending posttest ___/10

PHONEME/SOUND IDENTIFICATION

Initial Sound

Now we're going to listen for some sounds in words. First, I want you to tell me the beginning sound in the words I say. I want you to listen and tell me the sound you hear, not the letter that makes the sound. For example, the first (or beginning of) the word "sack" is /sss/. (*If a child responds with the letter name, tell him or her that you need to know the sound he or she hears and not the letter. Give him or her an additional chance to respond to the item.*) What is the first sound in the word . . . ?

Pretest		*Posttest*	
1. mat	_____	1. fit	_____
2. bed	_____	2. map	_____
3. soup	_____	3. book	_____
4. cap	_____	4. duck	_____

Final Sound

Now I want you to listen for the ending sound or the last sound in the words I say. For example, the last sound in the word "sack" is /k/. What is the last sound in the word . . . ?

5. fan	_____	5. gas	_____
6. rake	_____	6. ham	_____
7. leaf	_____	7. knot	_____
8. hot	_____	8. sick	_____

Total correct
   identification pretest ___/8

Total correct
   identification posttest ___/8

TOTAL PRETEST SCORE ___/26
(Rhyming + Blending + ID)

TOTAL POSTTEST SCORE ___/26
(Rhyming + Blending + ID)

The following sections of the test are *optional*. These sections evaluate phonics/sound–letter knowledge as well as phonemic awareness skills.

Grapheme–Phoneme (Letter–Sound)

Tell me a sound each of these letters make. (*Present the letter page on page 19, pointing to letters one at a time.*)

Pretest

1. m ____	6. a ____		
2. b ____	7. i ____		
3. z ____	8. u ____		
4. k ____	9. l ____		
5. n ____			

Posttest

1. m ____	6. a ____		
2. b ____	7. i ____		
3. z ____	8. u ____		
4. k ____	9. l ____		
5. n ____			

Phoneme–Grapheme (Sound–Letter)

Now I am going to say a sound, and I'd like you to write the letter that makes that sound. You can look at the alphabet written at the top of the page if you don't remember how to write a letter. (*Present short vowel sounds.*)

1. d ____	6. e ____	1. d ____	6. e ____
2. s ____	7. o ____	2. s ____	7. o ____
3. g ____	8. p ____	3. g ____	8. p ____
4. r ____	9. j ____	4. r ____	9. j ____
5. t ____	10. w ____	5. t ____	10. w ____

Total correct
   letter–sound pretest ___/19

Total correct
   letter–sound posttest ___/19

READING WORDS THAT CAN BE PHONETICALLY DECODED

Tell me what you think this word says. Many children your age can't read yet, but I just want you to take a guess about what the word might say. (*Reading list page included on page 20.*)

Pretest		*Posttest*	
1. fan	_____	1. kid	_____
2. run	_____	2. bus	_____
3. it	_____	3. at	_____
4. bag	_____	4. nut	_____
5. dad	_____	5. mom	_____

Total correct
    reading pretest ___/5

Total correct
    reading posttest ___/5

WRITING WORDS THAT CAN BE PHONETICALLY SEGMENTED

(*Give student a copy of the child's writing page located on page 18.*) Try to write the words I say. Listen for the sounds and write down the sounds that you hear. You can look at the alphabet at the top of your page if you forget how to write any of the letters. (*Score 1 point for each correct letter.*)

1. mad	_____	6. big	_____
2. nap	_____	7. sad	_____
3. bug	_____	8. man	_____
4. fun	_____	9. rug	_____
5. lip	_____	10. lid	_____

Total correct
    writing pretest ___/15

Total correct
    writing posttest ___/15

TOTAL OPTIONAL PRETEST ___/39   **TOTAL OPTIONAL POSTEST ___/39**

Child's Writing Page

(Copy page for pretest and posttest)

Child's name _____ Date _____

Teacher's name _____

Circle: Pretest sample   or   Posttest sample

Aa Bb Cc Dd Ee Ff Gg Hh Ii Jj Kk Ll Mm Nn Oo Pp Qq Rr Ss Tt Uu Vv Ww Xx Yy Zz

Sound–Letter

     1. _____

     2. _____

     3. _____

     4. _____

     5. _____

     6. _____

     7. _____

     8. _____

     9. _____

   10. _____

Writing Words

     1. _____

     2. _____

     3. _____

     4. _____

     5. _____

Letters for Grapheme–Phoneme (Letter–Sound) Assessment

m	b	z
k	n	a
i	u	l

Reading Lists

Chapter 3

The Whole-Class and Small-Group Lessons

Lesson 1: Concept of Words

Introduction

Preparation

- Copy reproducible pages for introduction.
- Cut apart word and picture cards.

Activity

Explain the concept of words:

- "Words mean something. We use words when we talk, and we use words when we read and write. When words are written on paper, there's a space between words."
- Show the first introduction card with multiple written words. First circle each word, then count the number of circles. Have children count written words looking for spaces without the teacher first circling words on the next two introduction cards:

  1. kitchen table (two words)
  2. big hat (two words)
  3. big black hat (three words)

- "When we change the words that we say or write, it changes what we mean. For example, this card says, 'Hickory dickory dock, the mouse ran up the clock.' First let's count the words in that sentence. (*Point to the words and count with class, nine words.*) Now we can change one of the words in the sentence and change what the sentence means. I'm going to cross out the word 'clock' and write 'tree' over it instead. Now let's read the sentence on the card again 'Hickory dickory dock the mouse ran up the tree.' Let's count the words again. There are still nine words, but now the mouse is running up a tree instead of a clock."
- Have children point out words that are written in the classroom (e.g., words on bulletin boards, names).

Discuss how words can be long or short.

- Play a guessing game to have the class decide which of the two words in the pictures is the longer word. As an example, show the class the picture of tape and explain that when we say the word "tape," it is a pretty short word. Show the picture of the lawnmower and say "When we say the word 'lawnmower,' it is a long word. We move our mouth a lot to say 'lawnmower.'" Ask two children to come to the front of the class. Have each child hold and name a picture. Have the class determine which child has the longer word of the following pairs of pictures:

  1. bug–octopus
  2. rope–grasshopper
  3. telephone–rake

4. van–watermelon
5. kangaroo–nose
6. light–elephant
7. ambulance–saw
8. banana–leaf

Literature

Introduce the book *The Itsy Bitsy Spider* by counting the number of words in the title. Read *The Itsy Bitsy Spider* by Iza Trapani.

- Point out words in the book that are long or short. For example, " 'waterspout' is a long word; 'out' is a short word; 'yellow' is a longer word than 'off.' "
- Talk about how many of the words rhyme or sound the same. Some examples include "pail–tail," "door–more," "chair–air," and "dry–try."

Whole-Class Activity

Have children sit in a circle: "We are going to say some nursery rhymes that we know, but each child will say one word of the nursery rhyme as we go around the circle. For example, if we did 'Little Boy Blue, come blow your horn,' Amanda (who is first in the circle) would say the word 'little,' Sam (who is sitting next to her) would say the word 'boy,' next Jacob would say the word 'blue.' "

- Use nursery rhymes or fingerplay words that your class knows. Other choices might include "Jack and Jill," "Little Miss Muffet," or "The Itsy Bitsy Spider."
- If some children have difficulty hearing word boundaries, you can explain that they said two words instead of one, or only said part of a word and not the whole word (if they said a syllable instead of a word).

Small-Group Activity

Preparation

- Copy the number strip.
- Copy and cut apart word cards.
- Place the number strip and the multiple-word cards included with this lesson in the middle of the small-group table.

Activity

- The children take turns picking a card from the top of the pile.
- Have them count how many words are on the card and then place that card under the corresponding number on the number strip. Continue until the cards run out.
- If a child says that "itsy bitsy spider" is two words, explain that it has three because "itsy" is a word, "bitsy" is a word, and "spider" is a word. You can circle the words and point to spaces between them if a child is having difficulty with the task.

Optional Related Activities

Ask the children to think of words that are very long.

- Have them bring back an item to school their parents thought was a long word and share it with the class.

Materials Needed

Reproducible materials accompanying the lesson:

- Introduction cards.
- Introduction pictures of short and long words.
- Number strip for the small-group activity.
- Eighteen multiple-word cards for the small-group activity.

Other materials:

- Book: *The Itsy Bitsy Spider* by Iza Trapani. New York: Scholastic, 1993. ISBN: 0-590-69821-4.

kitchen table

big hat

big black hat

Hickory dickory dock
the mouse ran up
the clock.

Introduction Pictures (Lesson 1)

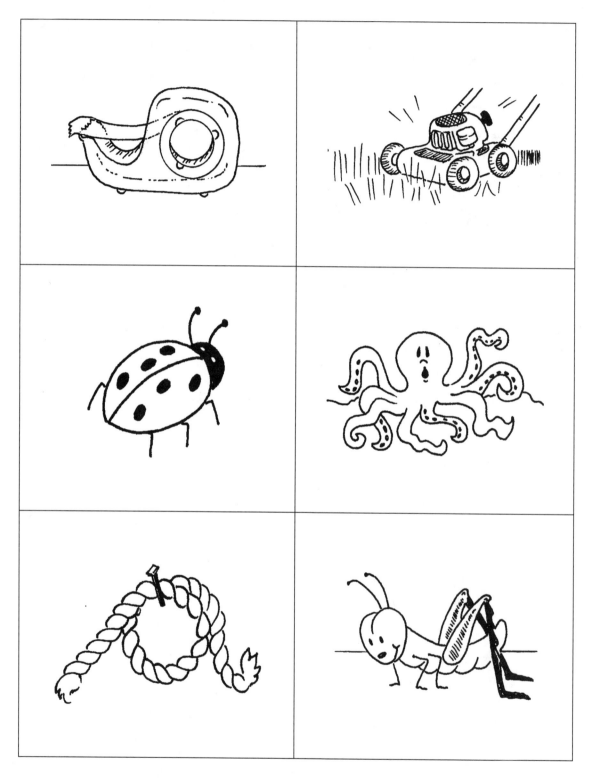

Introduction Pictures (Lesson 1)

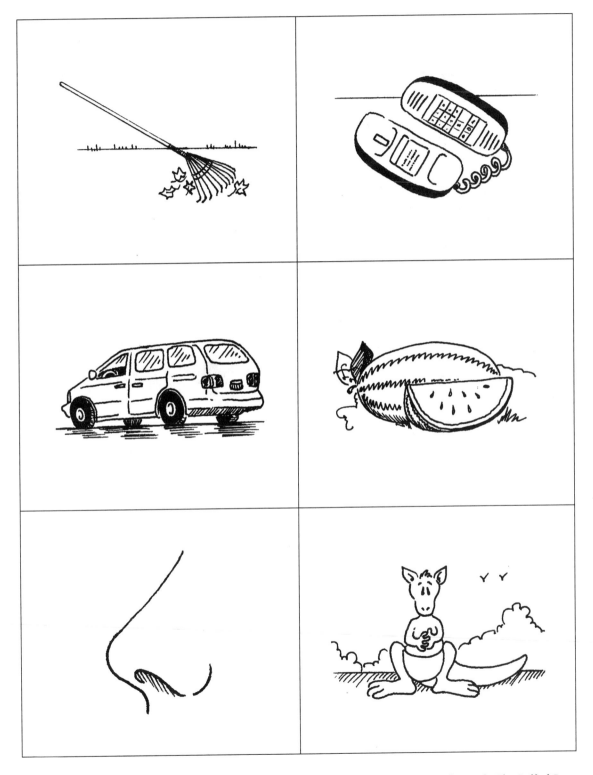

Introduction Pictures (Lesson 1)

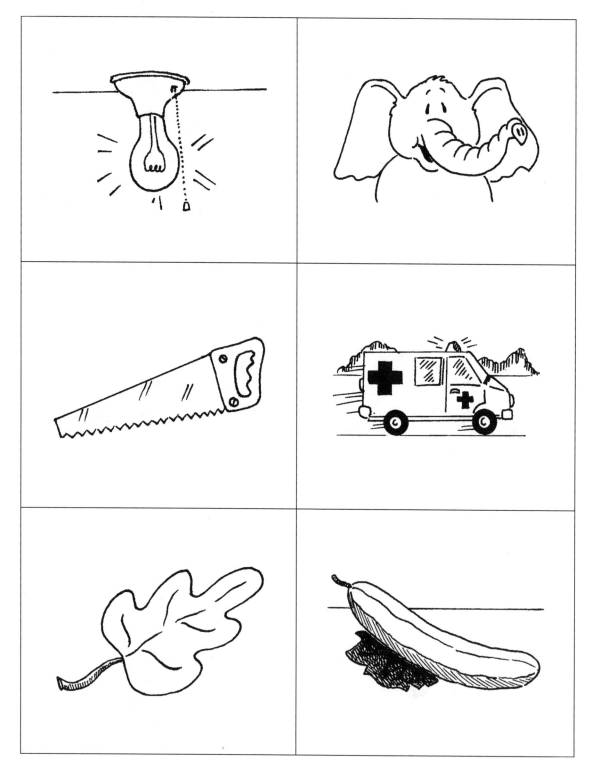

Small-Group Number Strip (Lesson 1)

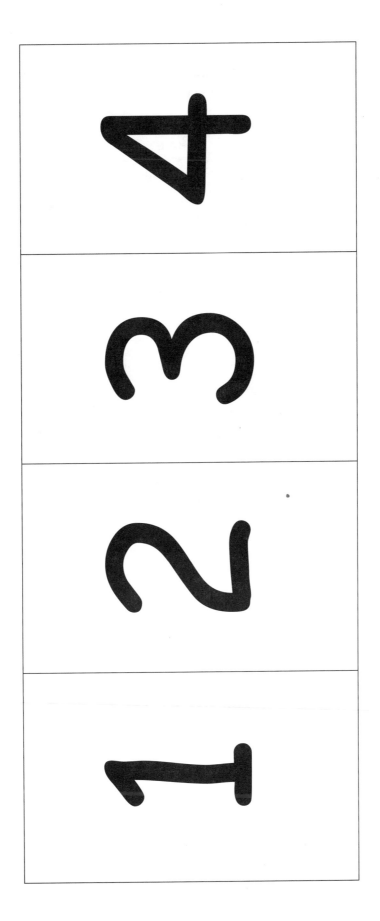

Small-Group Multiple-Word Cards (Lesson 1)

went the fan	chair	some dew
next to me	creep	up the yellow pail
was asleep	in the air	climbed up

Small-Group Multiple-Word Cards (Lesson 1)

out came the sun	fall	with his tail
down came the rain	mouse	out the door
maple tree	itsy bitsy spider	rocking chair

Lesson 2: Rhyme Recognition and Discrimination

Introduction

Preparation

- Gather objects for the same or different visual and auditory examples (e.g., pencils, ball, whistle, bell).

Activity

Discuss the concept of "same" as opposed to "different":

- "Two items can look the same when they have the same color and/or shape."
- Provide a visual example of items that are the "same," "alike," or "similar." For example, use two pencils and talk about their similarities (e.g., both are long, thin, and have erasers).
- Provide an example of similar sounds. Have the children close their eyes and blow a whistle two times. Ask them if the two sounds were alike.
- Provide a visual example of different objects. Explain how two objects such as a ball and a pencil are different.
- Provide an example of different sounds. Have the children close their eyes while you blow a whistle and a ring a bell. Ask them if the two sounds were similar or different.

Discuss the concept of rhymes

- "Words that rhyme are a little the same and a little different. When two words have the same ending sounds, they rhyme."
- Write two or three rhyming pairs of words on the board, underline the different part, and put a box around the same part. Use rhyming pairs that are spelled the same when using the written hints for when words rhyme (e.g., bat–mat, pig–big, *not* plane–train).
- Provide some rhyme discrimination examples. Ask the children to tell you if the two words rhyme:

  1. Sad–bad (rhyme)
  2. Mouse–house (rhyme)
  3. Hen–pen (rhyme)
  4. Boat–clock (do not rhyme). Explain how "oat" and "ock," the endings of boat–clock, don't sound the same; therefore, they do not rhyme.

Literature

Read *It's Raining, It's Pouring* by Kin Eagle.

- Point out how various pairs of words rhyme or do not rhyme after each verse (e.g., head/bed rhyme in first verse, sneezy/breezy rhyme in second verse, stars/easy do not rhyme, in second verse).

- After the first couple of verses, try to encourage class participation by asking the class if word pairs rhyme (e.g., ask the class if snowing/blowing rhyme after the third verse; also snowing/lunch, sunny/honey, fell/well, parts/Lindy, bed/head).
- If time and class attention allow, discuss other vocabulary/comprehension questions after the book. Sample questions include the following:

    1. "How did rain get in the man's house?"
    2. "What was the weather like when he was sneezing? How do you know?"
    3. "Why did the bees get angry?"
    4. "What is a well?"
    5. "What is the weather like in winter?"

Explain how we can talk about words in many different ways. Sometimes we talk about what words mean (e.g., "A well is something that holds water") and other times we think about how words sound (e.g., "Well and bell rhyme").

Whole-Class Activity

Preparation

- Gather a real umbrella, bucket, and box.
- Copy and cut apart the picture cards for whole-class activity. The teacher's rhyme cards are the cards on the left side of the page. The pictures on the right side of the page are for the children and should be placed in a box.

Activity

- Ask three children to come up in front of the class and have each take one picture from the box and hold it. The teacher, holding the open umbrella and a picture card, moves to each child and asks if the words depicted by the teacher's and child's pictures rhyme. If they rhyme, the child puts the teacher's card and his or her card in a bucket and the teacher gets a new picture from her (or his) pile. If the words represented by the pictures did not rhyme, the child puts his or her card back on the bottom of the stack of picture cards in the box. If the teacher's card did not match any of the children's cards, the teacher continues holding the same card as the next three children choose new pictures from the top of the children's stack in the box.
- Repeat until the cards or the children's attention are depleted.

Small Group

Preparation

- Copy reproducible materials (raindrop cards, umbrella picture) for small-group activity. Cut apart cards. A box is also needed for the activity.
- Place the picture of the umbrella in the middle of the small-group table. Place the cards with raindrops in a pile on the table.

Activity

- Each child takes a turn picking a card from the pile, naming the two pictures, and judging whether the names of the two pictures on the card rhyme. If they rhyme, the child places the card under the umbrella. If they do not rhyme, the card is placed in the box.
- If the child does not appear to understand the concept of rhyme, say the end of the words and ask if they sound alike (e.g., ail, ed). If the child still does not understand (and the rhyming portion is spelled the same), write down the words, say the end of each word, and put a box around the end of each word. Then, ask if they look alike and sound alike.

Optional Related Activities

- Call the children's names by producing a rhyme (e.g., " 'Jane/pane' rhymes, so line up now; 'Erin/book' does not rhyme, wait to line up").
- Read other literature with rhyming words.
- Home activity: Parents can play a memory game with children by cutting apart the pictures on a worksheet sent home (you can use picture pages from whole-class activity) and matching them by whether they rhyme.

Materials Needed

Reproducible materials accompanying the lesson:

- 18 picture cards for whole-class activity.
- Picture of umbrella for small-group activity.
- 18 raindrop picture cards for the small group.

Other materials:

- Book *It's Raining, It's Pouring* by Kin Eagle. Dallas, TX: Whispering Coyote Press, 1994. ISBN: 1-879085-71-2.
- Umbrella for whole-class activity.
- Bucket for whole-class activity.
- Box for whole-class activity and small-group activity.
- Pencils for the introduction.
- Whistle for the introduction.
- Bell or other noisemaker for the introduction.
- Ball for the introduction.

Whole-Class Activity Pictures (Lesson 2)

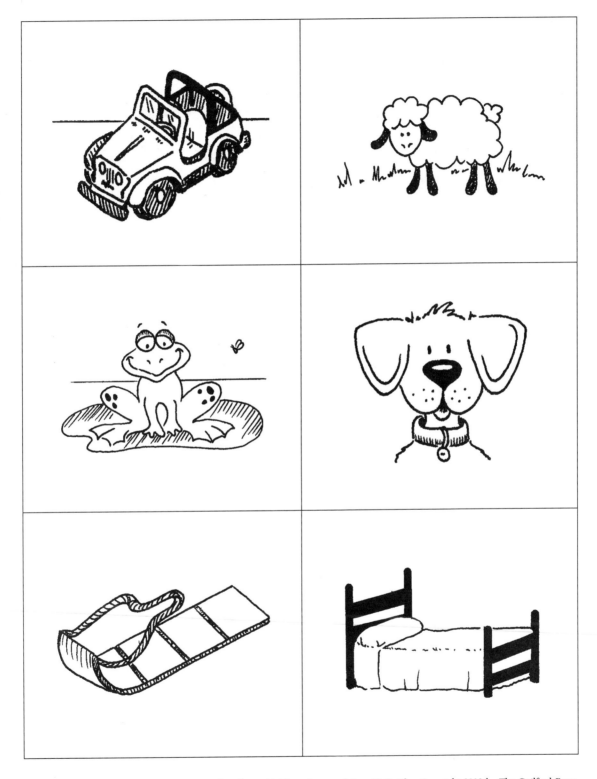

Whole-Class Activity Pictures (Lesson 2)

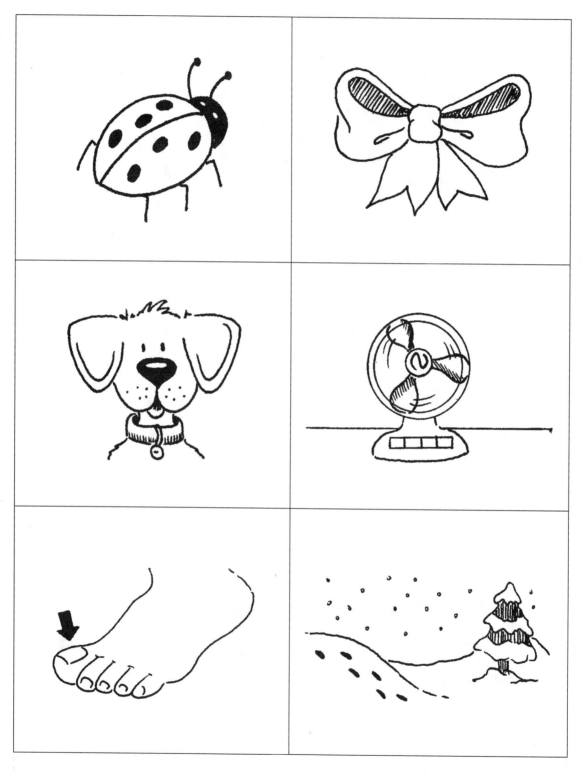

Whole-Class Activity Pictures (Lesson 2)

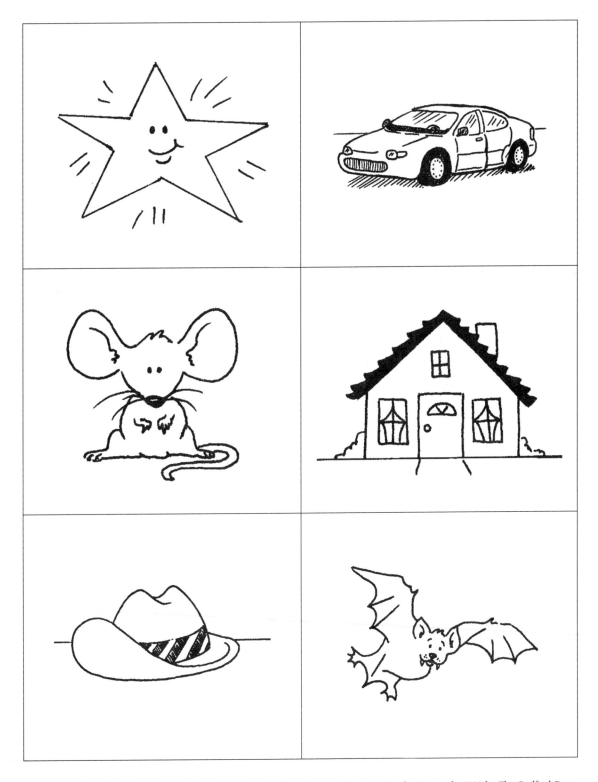

Small-Group Pictures (Lesson 2)

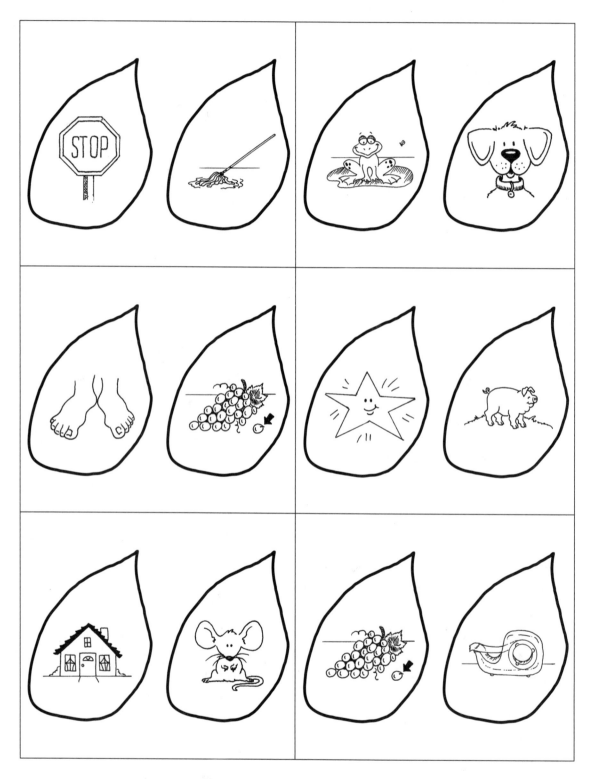

Small-Group Pictures (Lesson 2)

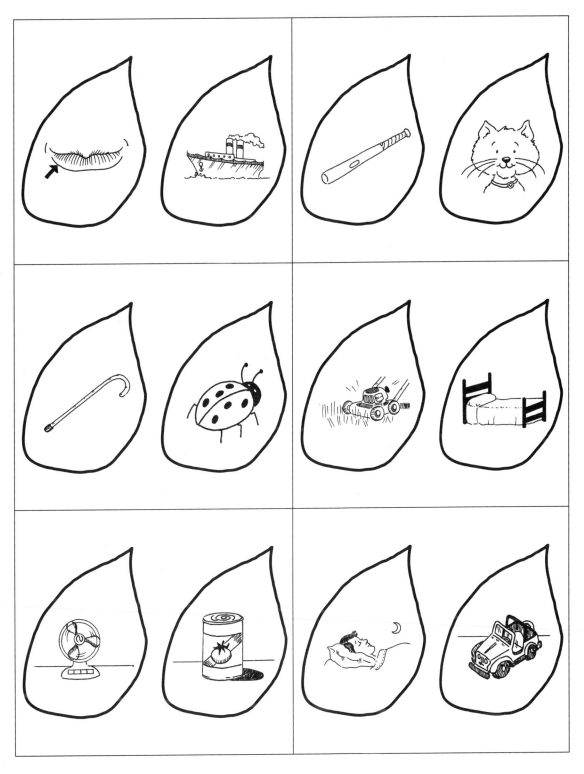

Small-Group Pictures (Lesson 2)

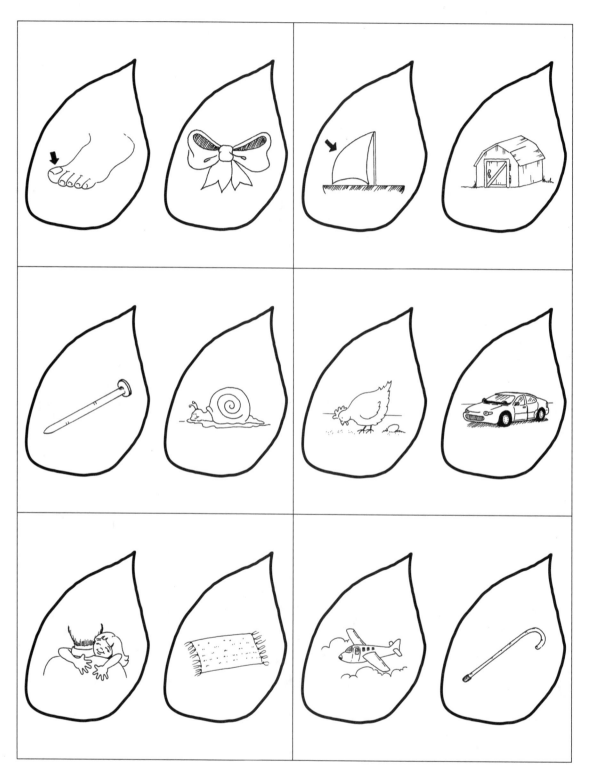

Small-Group Pictures (Lesson 2)

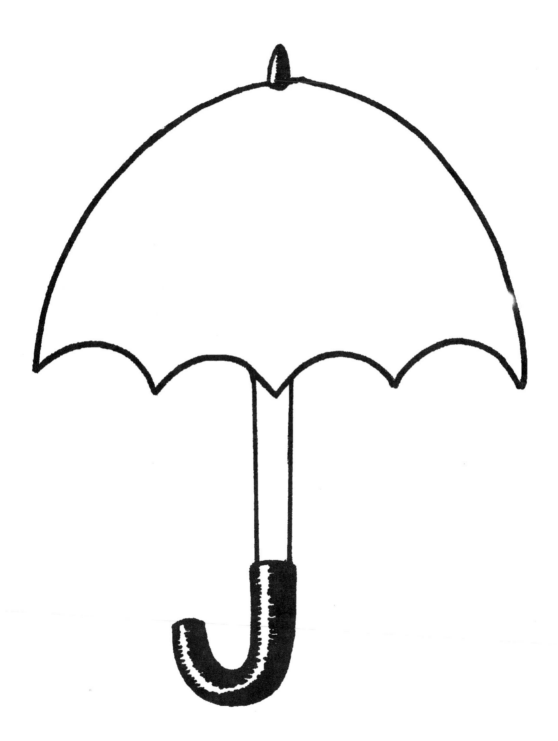

Lesson 3: Rhyme Choice

Introduction

Preparation

- Copy introduction picture pages.

Activity

Review the concept of rhyme.

- "When words rhyme, the ends of words sound the same but the beginning sound is different."

Review rhyme discrimination.

- Ask the class to listen and tell you if these words rhyme or not:
  1. "Tall–ball (*pause*); that's right, they rhyme. We hear 'all' at the end of both words."
  2. "Run–sun (*pause*); yes, they rhyme. We hear 'un' at the end of both words."
  3. "Sit–can (*pause*); they do not rhyme. The ends of the words don't sound the same: 'it–an.'"
  4. "Wing–sing (*pause*); they rhyme. We hear 'ing' at the end of both words."
  5. "Duck–luck (*pause*); they rhyme. We hear 'uck' at the end of both words."
  6. "Red–chair (*pause*); they do not rhyme. The ends of the words do not sound the same: 'ed–air.'"

Ask the children to find the two rhyming words represented by each of the three large pictures.

- Ask one child to come to the front of the class and show the first page of introduction pictures. Name the three pictures for the child. Have the child choose the two pictures that rhyme. Continue activity with the five other introductory pages.
  1. bow–toe–dog
  2. house–cat–bat
  3. frog– star–dog
  4. jar–car–mop
  5. rain–bed–train
  6. rug–pan–van

Literature

Read *Five Little Ducks* by Pamela Paparone.

- Review the concept of "words" by counting the number of words in the title of the book.
- The book contains a lot of repetition, so you can point to the words and the children can finish the repetitive phrases (e.g., "Over the hills and _____ [far away]").
- Point out rhyming words in book (e.g., day–away, quack–back).

Whole-Class Activity

Preparation

- Make "duck pond" on floor with string/rope/tape or use a small plastic pool.
- Copy and cut apart all three pages of small ducks. Place all small ducks in the "pond."

Activity

- Ask two children to come up at a time, and have each child pick a duck from the pond.
- They will decide if the words depicted by the drawings on their two ducks rhyme.
- If they rhyme, they will hand the cards to the teacher.
- If they don't rhyme, ask them to produce a word that rhymes with their picture.
- If they are unable to produce a rhyming word, they can call on another child to help.
- Replace nonrhyming cards back into pond. Call on the next two children.

Small-Group Activity

Preparation

- Copy and cut apart mother ducks.
- Place each of the three big mother ducks and the pile of 15 little baby ducks (the two pages labeled whole class and small group) in the center of the table.
- The pictures on the mother ducks and the baby ducks make up three different rhyme families.

Activity

- Name the pictures on the mother ducks ("bow, nail, mop").
- Explain to the children that they will draw a card from the pile and then find which mother duck rhymes with their picture.
- Once the child locates the mother duck/rhyming family, he or she places the baby duck under the mother duck and names the rhyming pictures.
- Continue the activity in a similar manner with the other children.
- Teaching for those children who do not understand:

1. Repeat words together; emphasize the ending sounds.
2. If they still do not understand, divide the initial sound or sound cluster from the rest of the word when repeating the two words and then question if the words rhyme (i.e., "tr—ail, n—ail: Do you hear 'ail' at the ends of both of them? Then they rhyme. Tr—ail, b—ow: Do you hear 'ail' at the end of both of those words? The ends of the words are different, 'ail'–'ow.' They don't rhyme.")

Other Related Activities

- Call on children for other tasks during the week (when several children have their hands raised) by using words (real or nonsense) that rhyme with their names (e.g., "If your name rhymes with 'wacob,' I would like you to answer; if your name rhymes with 'games,' you should answer"; and so on).

- Play "I spy" with rhyming words (e.g., the teacher looks at a box and says, "I spy something that rhymes with 'fox'"; then looks at a book and says "I spy something that rhymes with 'shook'"; and so on).
- Teach "Five Little Ducks" with hand motions. If time allows, act out fingerplay with five children in front of the whole class. During these activities, have the children say the rhyming words. Point out the rhyming words (e.g., "quack–back").

Materials Needed

Reproducible materials accompanying the lesson:

- Large pictures for the introduction (six pages).
- 14 baby ducks from the small group plus 9 more baby ducks for the whole-class duck pond (all three pages of small ducks).
- Pictures of 3 mother ducks and 14 baby ducks for the small group (two pages of small ducks).

Other materials:

- Book: *Five Little Ducks* by Pamela Paparone. New York: Scholastic, 1995. ISBN: 0-590-96581-6.
- String, rope, tape, or swimming pool to make the "duck pond" on the floor.

Introduction Pictures (Lesson 3)

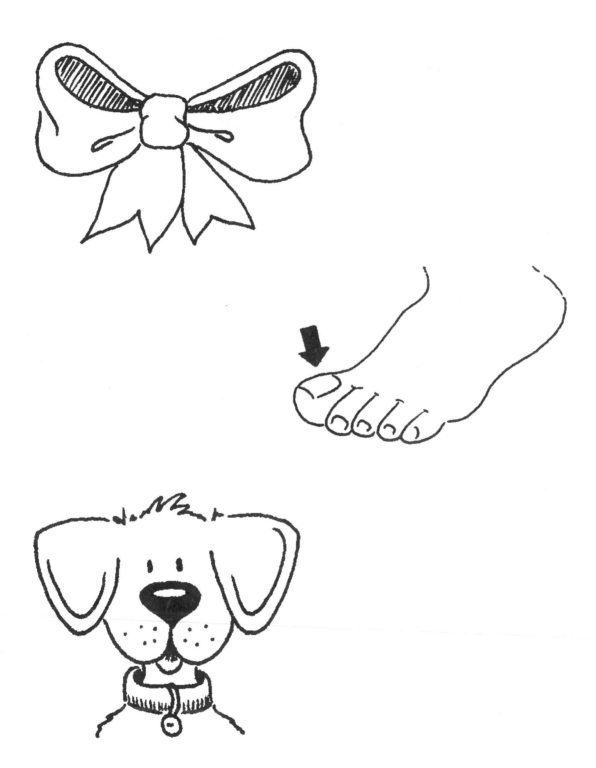

Introduction Pictures (Lesson 3)

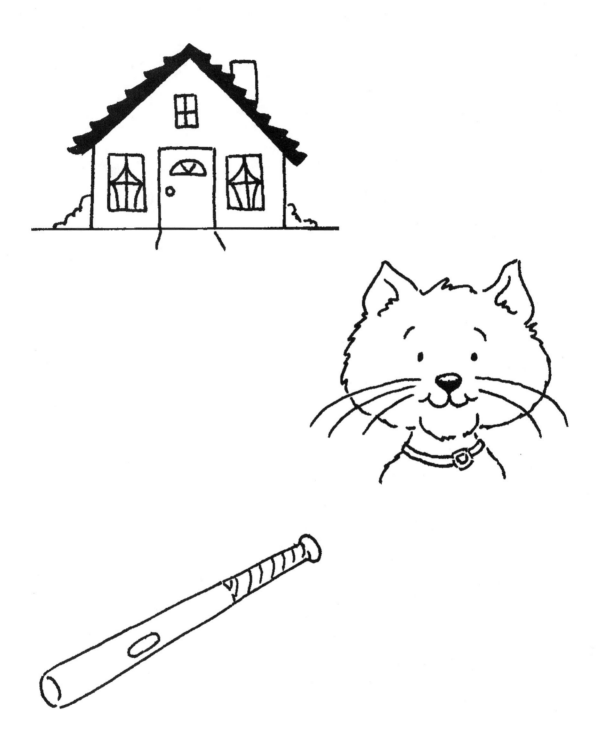

Introduction Pictures (Lesson 3)

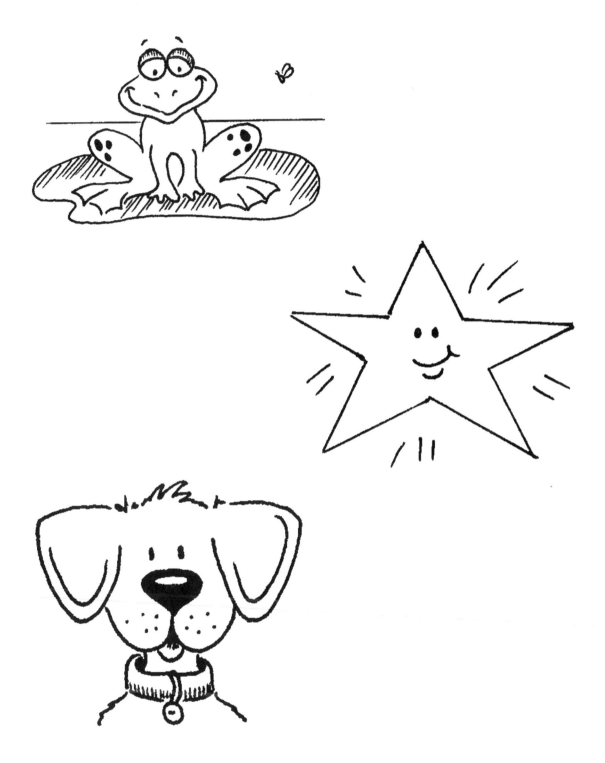

Introduction Pictures (Lesson 3)

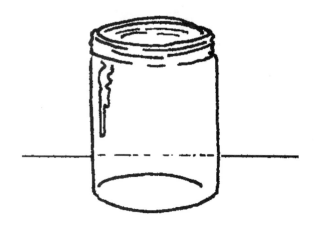

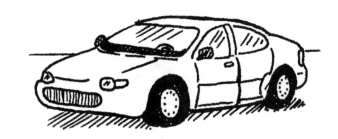

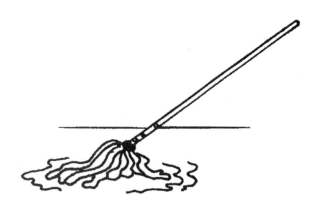

Introduction Pictures (Lesson 3)

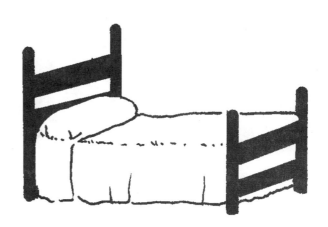

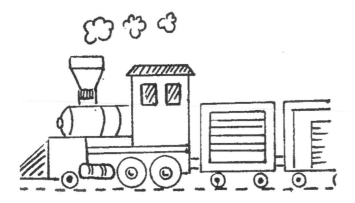

Introduction Pictures (Lesson 3)

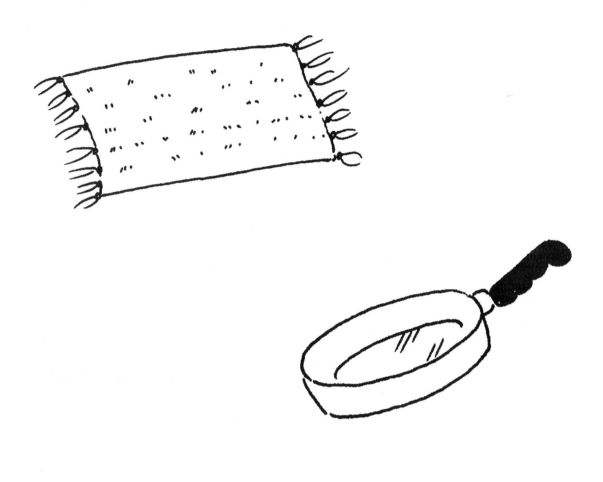

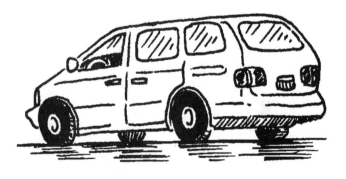

Pictures for the Whole Class
(can-man-fan-pan-van, lip-ship-rip-chip/dip) (Lesson 3)

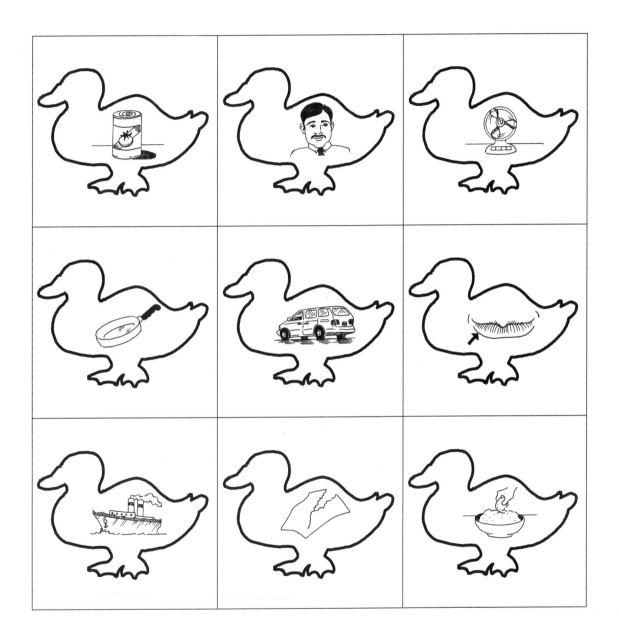

Pictures for the Whole Class and the Small Group
(toe-snow-mow-crow, top-pop-stop-shop) (Lesson 3)

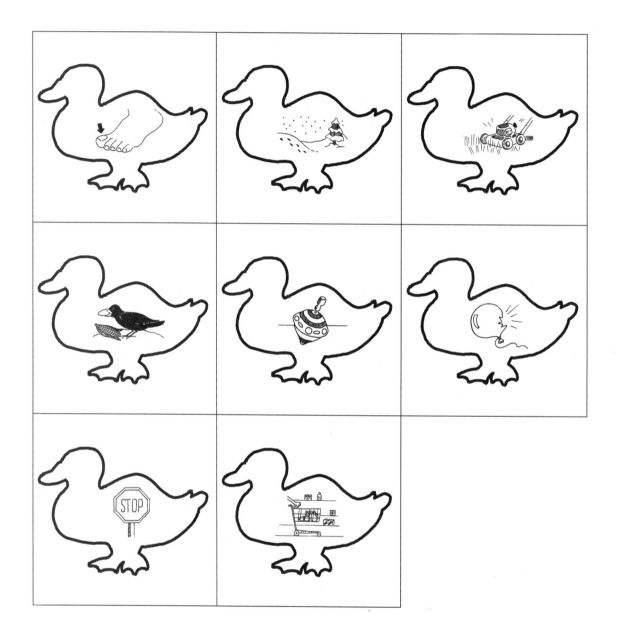

Pictures for the Whole Class and the Small Group
(trail-tail-snail-sail-whale-mail) (Lesson 3)

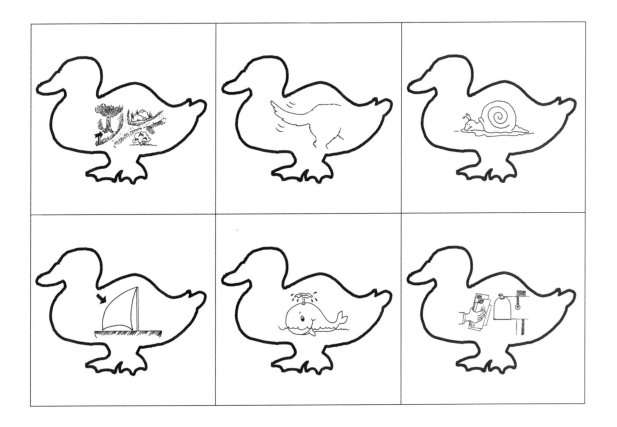

Pictures for the Small-Group Activity: "Mother Ducks" (Lesson 3)

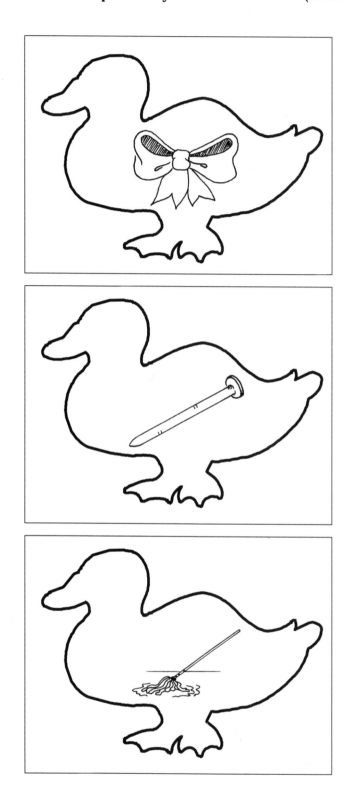

Lesson 4: Rhyme Production

Introduction

The teacher: "We have been talking about rhyming words. This week we're going to be thinking of more words that rhyme or sound alike at the end."

- "Let's start with some nursery rhymes that you probably know. Nursery rhymes often have many rhyming words in them. When I say part of the nursery rhyme, I'll leave some rhyming words out that you as a class can fill in and say for me."

  1. Hickory dickory dock, the mouse ran up the _____ (clock). Explain, "That's right. 'Clock' finishes that sentence and 'dock' and 'clock' rhyme."
  2. Little Bo Peep lost her _____ (sheep). "Which of the words that I said rhymes with 'sheep'?" (peep)
  3. Twinkle, twinkle, little star, how I wonder where you _____ (are). "Which word that I said rhymes with 'are'?" (star)
  4. Jack and Jill went up a _____ (hill). "Which word rhymed with 'hill'?" (Jill)
  5. Humpty Dumpty sat on a wall, Humpty Dumpty had a great _____ (fall). "Which word rhymed with 'fall'?" (wall)
  6. Little Boy Blue come blow your horn, the sheep's in the meadow, the cow's in the _____ (corn). "Which word rhymed with 'corn'?" (horn)

Literature

Read several nursery rhymes from any Mother Goose rhyme book.

- Point out rhyming words to class at times (e.g., "'Dock' and 'clock' sound the same at the end—they rhyme").
- Pause during reading and let children fill in rhyming words (e.g., "Humpty Dumpty sat on a wall, Humpty Dumpty had a great _____"; pause for the class to fill in "fall").

Whole-Class Activity

The whole-class activity consists of singing the "Itsy Bitsy Spider" song and thinking of other words that rhyme with rhyming words in the song. You read the book *The Itsy Bitsy Spider*, as told and illustrated by Iza Trapani in Lesson 1. You may wish to read the book again today before singing the song, or you may wish to show the pictures from the book to help the class remember the words of the song while singing.

- Sing verse 1 of the "Itsy Bitsy Spider" with class as a whole and do fingerplay actions with the song.
- The rhyming words in the first verse are "spout–out." "Who can think of some other real or made-up words that rhyme with 'spout' and 'out'?" (real words: shout, pout, stout; made-up words: cout, tout, lout, fout, sout, wout, mout, nout, dout, jout, vout, etc.)

- Sing each verse as you're showing the class the pictures in the book for that verse. After verse 2 has been sung, explain that the rhyming words in the verse were "wall–fall" and "blow–go." Choose a child to say another word (real or made up) that rhymes with "wall–fall." Then call on two more children to think of other words that can rhyme with "wall–fall." Next choose three children to each think of other words that rhyme with "blow–go."
- Repeat singing and thinking of rhymes for each of the verses 3–6.
- Rhyming words:

    1. Verse 3, pail–tail, door–more
    2. Verse 4, chair–air, asleep–creep
    3. Verse 5, tree–me, dry–try
    4. Verse 6, stop–top, done–sun

Small-Group Activity

Preparation

- Copy pages with sentences at the top. (Make a copy of each of the three pages for every child in the group.)

Activity

Explain to the children that they are each going to make some new rhymes that change the words in some of the nursery rhymes we know.

- The teacher reads the original rhyme and points to words in written sentences.
- Discuss the rhyming words in the original rhyme.
- The teacher then reads the new sentences and asks the child to think of a word that rhymes with the underlined word.
- The teacher writes the rhyming word on the child's paper.
- The child can draw a picture to depict the old and new rhymes.

Optional Related Activities

- Read other rhyming books. Emphasize the first word of a rhyme pair; let the class guess/fill in the second word of the rhyme pair during book readings.
- Ask children to make up a silly word that rhymes with their name (e.g., Jacob—wacob, macob, facob, and the like).

Materials Needed

Reproducible materials accompanying the lesson:

- Copy new nursery rhyme pages for each child in the small group.

Other materials:

- Book: Any Mother Goose rhyme book. One good choice might be *Hey Diddle Diddle and Other Mother Goose Rhymes* by Tomie dePaola. New York: Putnam, 1988. ISBN: 88-11561.
- Book: *The Itsy Bitsy Spider,* as told and illustrated by Iza Trapani. New York: Scholastic, 1993. ISBN: 0-590-69821-4.

Hickory Dickory Dock
the mouse ran up the clock.

Hickory Dickory <u>Dee</u>
the mouse ran up the _____.

Jack and Jill
went up the hill.

Jack and <u>Jane</u>
rode on a _____.

Little Boy Blue
come blow your horn
the sheep s in the meadow
the cow s in the corn.

Little Boy Blue
wake up <u>quick</u>.
The sheep and cow aren t feeling well
they re really quite _____.

Lesson 5: Syllable Counting

Introduction

Explain syllable counting:

- "Today we're going to listen to words. Some words are long and have many syllables or beats in them. Other words are shorter and only have one or two syllables or beats in them. A syllable is a part of a word. We can hear syllables in words and clap once for each syllable."
- "Let's do some syllable clapping and counting."

  1. snow(*clap*)man(*clap*). (*Clap as you say each syllable*.) "We clapped two times as I said 'snowman.' There are two syllables in the word 'snowman.'"
  2. mock(*clap*)ing(*clap*)bird(*clap*). "How many times did we clap as I said mockingbird? We clapped three times. There are three syllables in the word mockingbird."
  3. rat(*clap*)tle(*clap*)snake(*clap*). "How many claps or syllables were there for 'rattlesnake'?"
  4. rock(*clap*). "Rock is a short word. We just clapped one time. There's just one syllable in the word 'rock.'"
  5. chalk(*clap*)board(*clap*). "How many syllables are in the word 'chalkboard'?"
  6. drag(*clap*)on(*clap*)fly(*clap*). "How many syllables in the word 'dragonfly'?"

Explain that you will now say a word and have the children clap to count the syllables. "Now I'm just going to say the word and not clap."

- "I'll call on one of you. Your job is to say the word that I said. Clap once for each syllable or beat in the word as you say it."

  1. raindrop. "You say 'raindrop' and clap once as you say each syllable. Good, you clapped two times as you said 'raindrop.' There are two syllables in the word 'raindrop.'"
  2. grasshopper (*child says word and claps*). "I heard three claps. There must be three syllables in the word 'grasshopper.'"
  3. jar (1 syllable)
  4. elevator (4 syllables)
  5. blacktop (2 syllables)
  6. flowerpot (3 syllables)

Literature

Read *Guess How Much I Love You* by Sam McBratney. Read the first page.

- After reading the page, count and clap syllables in the following words:

  1. little (2)
  2. nutbrown (2)
  3. bed (1)

- Also discuss the meaning of the word "hare." "Hare is another name for rabbit. How many syllables are there in the word 'hare'? How many syllables are there in the word 'rabbit'?"
- After reading the third page, count the number of syllables in the word "stretching" (2).
- Other words from the book with which you can practice counting syllables during or after the book reading include the following:

1. love (1)
2. high (1)
3. idea (3)
4. toes (1)
5. bouncing (2)
6. hop (1)
7. hopping (2)
8. sleepy (2)

Whole-Class Activity

Preparation

- Place four green towels on the floor approximately 1 foot apart.

Activity

"We just read a book about two rabbits. Real rabbits don't walk or run, they hop or jump."

- "For our next activity each of you will get to pretend to be a rabbit. I have four green towels on the floor with a little bit of space between each of the towels. We are going to pretend the green towels are bushes. When it's your turn to be a rabbit, I'll tell you a word. You say the word that I say. Tell me how many syllables are in the word. Clap as you say the word to figure out how many syllables there are. Next, you get to jump into the bushes, once for each syllable in the word. If there are two syllables in the word (e.g., 'birthday'), you will jump to the first bush (for the first syllable, 'birth'), then to the second bush (for the second syllable, 'day'). If there are four syllables, you will jump four times all the way to the last bush."
- Words for whole-class activity:

1. snowflake (2)
2. tablespoon (3)
3. announcement (3)
4. grandpa (2)
5. mailbox (2)
6. flag (1)
7. bookkeeper (3)
8. graduation (4)
9. tugboat (2)
10. grandmother (3)
11. fisherman (3)

12. policewoman (4)
13. afternoon (3)
14. swing (1)
15. Cinderella (4)
16. mouse (1)
17. supermarket (4)
18. happy (2)
19. basket (2)
20. parachute (3)
21. arrow (2)
22. Saturday (3)
23. skateboard (2)

Small-Group Activity

Preparation for the Bunny Rabbit Race

- Choose as many colors of construction paper as you have children in your small group. Cut 10 circles out of each color. Arrange each set of circles in a straight line next to each other on a table or floor. This will be the rabbit race track. Place a bunny cutout on top of the first circle of each color, and place a string or piece of yarn straight across between the ninth and tenth circles of each color. The string is the finish line.
- Copy and cut up picture cards for small group, mix up, and place face down in front of teacher at table or on floor.

Activity

- Explain to the children that each of them will be a bunny who is running a race. They will take turns drawing a card from the pile. Each child will say the word on the picture and then figure out how many syllables are in the word. The child will then move his or her bunny forward one hop for each syllable in the word. The first bunny to cross the finish line at the end wins. You can repeat this game as often as time and the children's attention permits.
- If a child is having difficulty determining the number of syllables in words, you can clap with the child as he or she says the word. You may also wish to say the word for the child, pausing slightly between each syllable as a hint for him or her to clap. You might practice putting up a finger each time a syllable is said in a word; then at the end of the word the child can count the number of fingers that are up to determine the number of syllables.

Optional Related Activities

Read *The Grouchy Ladybug* by Eric Carle. Hong Kong: Harper Trophy, 1977. ISBN: 0-06-443116-9.

- Count the number of syllables for each animal the ladybug asks to fight.
- As an alternative similar book, you could use *The Very Lazy Ladybug* by Isobel Finn and Jack

Tickle. Alpharetta, GA: Tiger Tales, 2001. ISBN: 1-58-825007-9. Count the number of syllables for each animal or place the ladybug tries to sleep on.

- Ask the children to count the number of syllables in their last name.
- Count the number of syllables in equipment or materials as you hand them out for playtime.

Materials Needed

Reproducible materials accompanying the lesson:

- Rabbit cutout for each child in the small group.
- Colored circles to arrange on the table for each rabbit track in the small group (10 circles in one color for each child in the group).
- Picture cards for the small group.

Other materials:

- Book: *Guess How Much I Love You* by Sam McBratney. New York: Scholastic, 1994. ISBN: 0-590-67981-3.
- Four green towels for whole-class bushes.
- String/yarn to lay across last circles on the small-group rabbit track for the finish line.

Small-Group Pictures (Lesson 5)

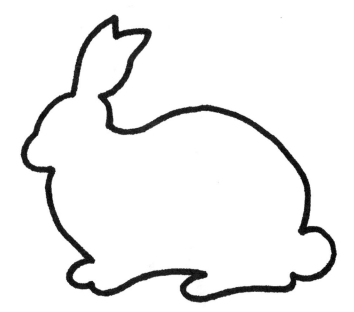

Small-group rabbit pattern.

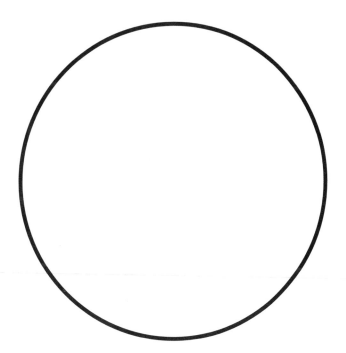

Circle pattern for the bunny rabbit racetrack game board. Trace and cut out 10 circles on each color construction paper. You'll need one color (group of 10 circles) for each child in the small group.

Small-Group Pictures (Lesson 5)

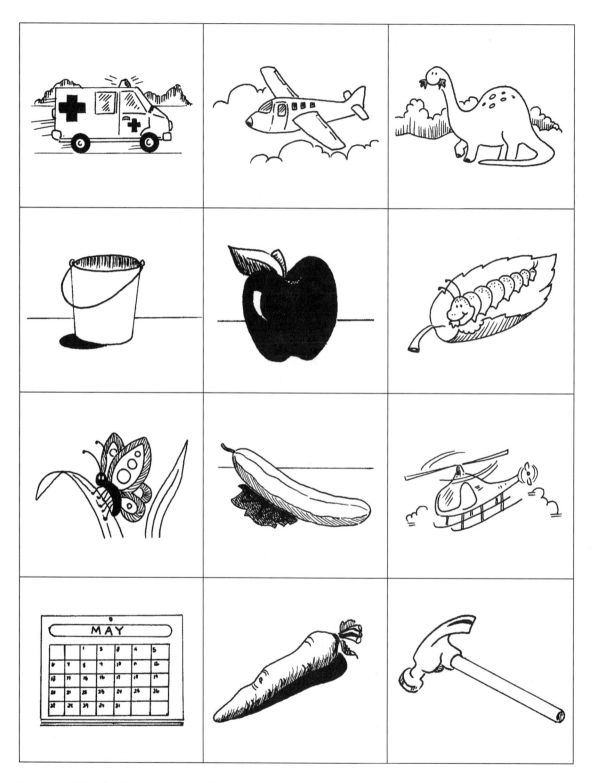

Small-Group Pictures (Lesson 5)

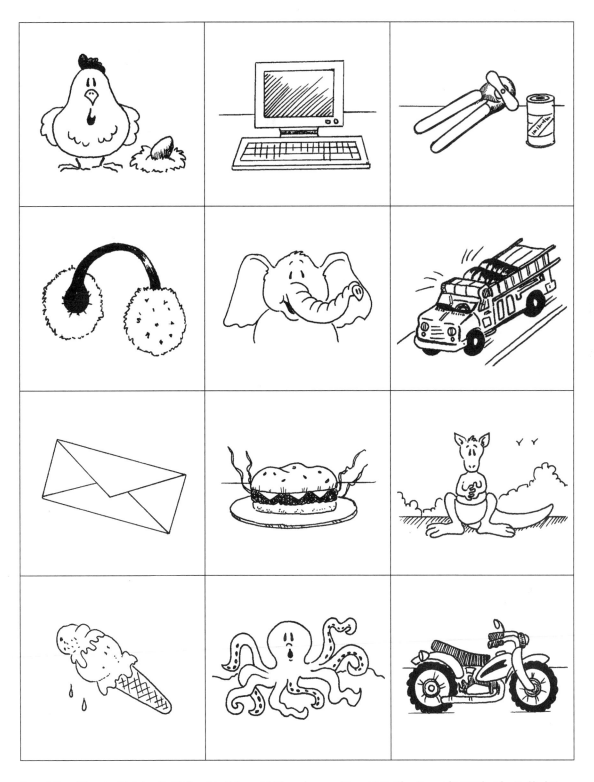

Small-Group Pictures (Lesson 5)

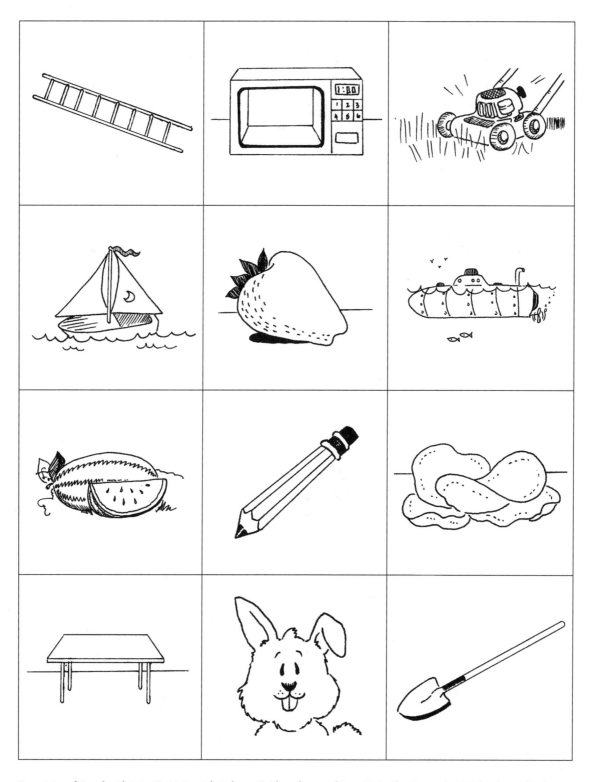

Lesson 6: Syllable Blending

Introduction

Review syllable counting.

- Have children count syllables by holding up a finger for each syllable as you say the following words:

  1. seesaw
  2. basketball
  3. earring
  4. bear
  5. bookmark

Explain syllable blending:

- "Now you are going to listen to the parts of words or syllables. You are going to have to remember the syllables and put them together to figure out the word."

Play a guessing game:

- "I'm thinking of some kinds of food. I'm going to say the words in parts; then you have to put the syllables together to guess what I'm thinking of." Pause approximately 1–2 seconds between syllables. You may wish to begin with a short pause at the beginning and lengthen the pause as the class becomes more proficient with the task.

  1. po—ta—to
  2. straw—ber("bear")—ry
  3. pea—nut
  4. wa—ter—mel—on
  5. ap—ple
  6. ham—burg—er
  7. mac—a—ro—ni
  8. pop—corn

Literature

Preparation

- Popcorn snack for children as they listen to popcorn book (optional)

Read *The Popcorn Shop* by Alice Low, and have children recall events from the book when the book is finished.

- "Let's try to remember some of the things that Nell made out of popcorn. I'll say the words slowly, and you raise your hand if you know what word or words I am saying: Some food Nell made from popcorn was . . . "

1. pan—cakes
2. pick—les
3. Pop—si—cles

- "Now let's try to remember some of the places the popcorn went when the popcorn machine made too much popcorn. The popcorn was in . . . "

1. bar—ber—chair
2. scare—crow—clothes
3. fire—truck—hose
4. pump—kin—patch

Whole-Class Activity

Preparation

- Set up some type of barrier (e.g., shelves or a table) for children to crouch behind during the activity before "popping up" to be popcorn.

Activity

- "We are going to take turns being popcorn. I will ask two or three children to come up and stand behind the (shelves/table/some type of barrier). I will tell each child who is up in front being the popcorn one syllable from a word. Then one at a time, they will each pop up and say the syllable that I told them. The rest of the class needs to listen very carefully and try to figure out the secret words the popcorn kids say. After each word, I'll choose new children to come up front so that everyone will get a turn being popcorn."
- Words for the whole-class activity:

1. sail-boat (Whisper "sail" in the first child's ear and "boat" in the second child's ear. Instruct the two children to squat down behind the barrier. Have the first child pop up [stand up] and say his or her syllable, then immediately have the second child do the same. Call on someone in the class to guess what word was said.)
2. bath-tub
3. base-ball
4. cow-boy-hat
5. birth-day
6. bum-ble-bee
7. air-plane
8. lawn-mow-er
9. pa-per
10. Mon-day
11. el-e-phant
12. ti-ger

13. bi-cy-cle
14. spi-der
15. tel-e-phone

Small-Group Activity

Preparation

- Copy bingo cards.
- Copy and cut up word-card page, mix up the cards, and place them face down in front of you on the small-group table.
- Popcorn or other bingo markers are also needed.

Activity

- Give each child a different bingo card.
- Explain to the children that you are going to take a word off of your pile and say the word in pieces or syllables.
- The children need to listen to the syllables and decide if they have a picture of the word you say in pieces on their card.
- If they have a picture of the word you say on their card, they can put a piece of popcorn on the picture.
- The first child with all of the pictures covered with popcorn wins.
- You can repeat this game as often as time and the group's attention permits.
- If a child is having difficulty determining words that you are saying with pauses between the syllable, you can repeat the syllables with a shorter pause between the syllables or you can tell the child what category the word is from (e.g., "It's a type of food," or "It's a type of animal [or clothes, etc.]"). You can also have the child repeat each syllable after you say it, then ask the child to say the syllables quickly together.

Optional Related Activities

- Call on children to line up and participate in activities by pausing between syllables in either the children's first or last names throughout the week.
- Have children guess what they are having for snacks or lunch by pausing between syllables of names of food.

Materials Needed

Reproducible materials accompanying the lesson:

- Bingo cards for the small-group activity.
- Word cards cut apart for the small-group bingo game.

Other materials:

- Book: *The Popcorn Shop* by Alice Low. New York: Scholastic, 1993. ISBN: 0-590-4721-X
- Popcorn.
- Cups to hold the popcorn.
- Popcorn for bingo markers in the small-group activity.

Small-Group Bingo Card (Lesson 6)

POPCORN BINGO

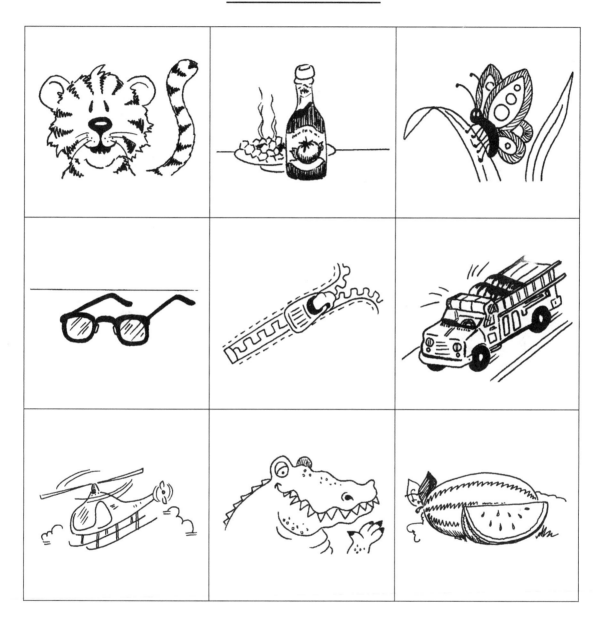

Small-Group Bingo Card (Lesson 6)

POPCORN BINGO

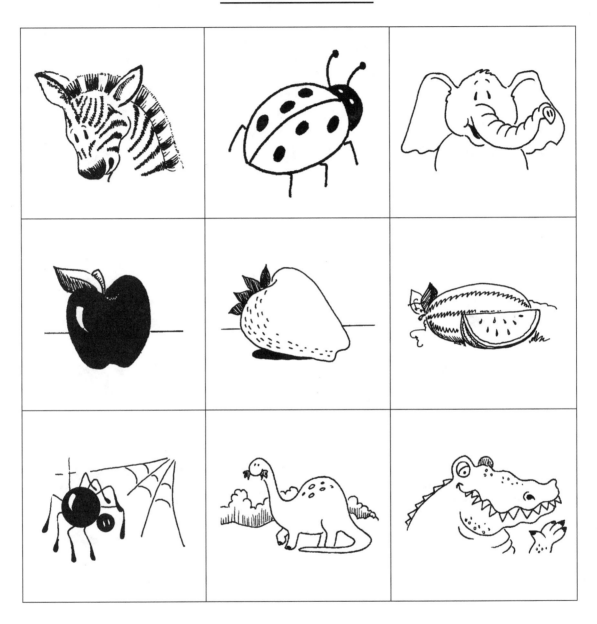

Small-Group Bingo Card (Lesson 6)

POPCORN BINGO

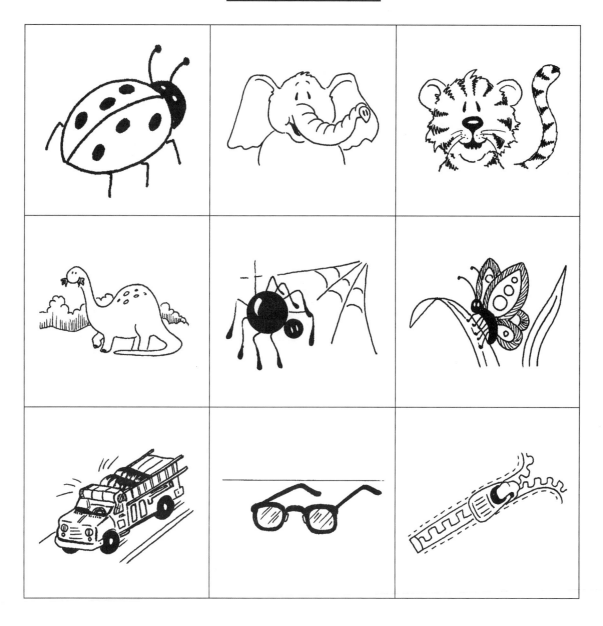

Small-Group Bingo Card (Lesson 6)

POPCORN BINGO

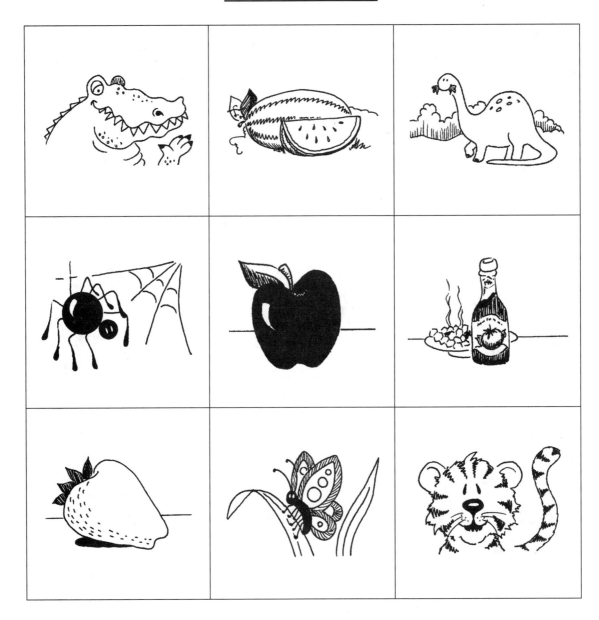

Small-Group Bingo Card (Lesson 6)

POPCORN BINGO

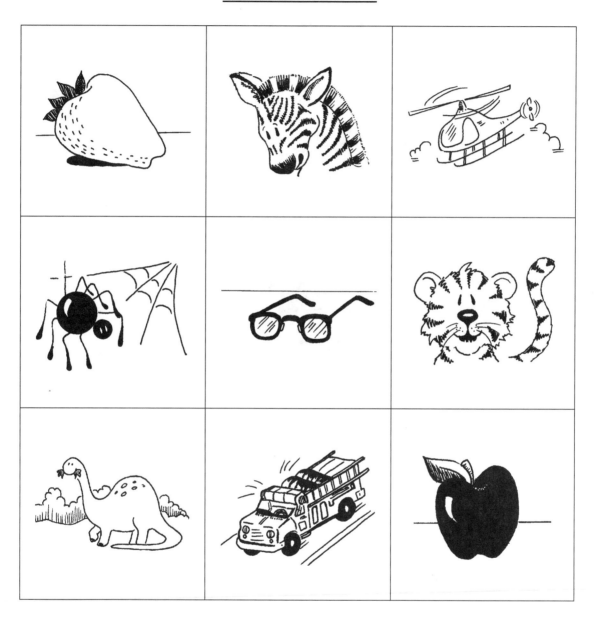

Small-Group Bingo Card (Lesson 6)

POPCORN BINGO

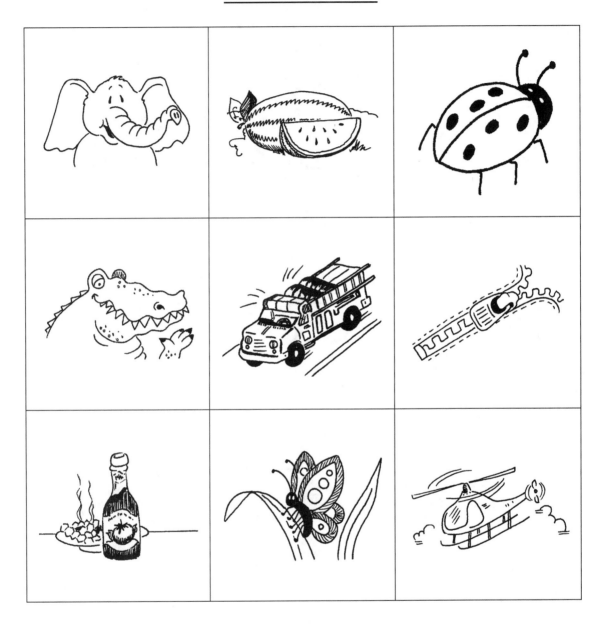

Small-Group Word Cards for Teacher to Draw from the Pile for Popcorn Bingo (Lesson 6)

ti-ger	el-e-phant	la-dy-bug	ze-bra
ketch-up	ap-ple	straw-ber-ry	wa-ter-mel-on
but-ter-fly	spi-der	di-no-saur	al-li-ga-tor
glass-es	zip-per	fire-truck	hel-i-cop-ter

Lesson 7: Syllable Deletion

Introduction

The teacher: "Today we're going to talk about taking parts of words away. We'll listen to a long word, then we'll take away one of the syllables and try to figure out what parts of the word are left without that syllable. Lets say a word together and put up a finger each time we hear a syllable."

- "See" (*first finger up*) "saw" (*second finger up*). "How many syllables were in the word 'see-saw'? That's right, two. Now what part of the word would be left if we took away 'saw' (*put second finger down*). All that would be left is just the 'see' part of the word."
- "Let's do another one. Put your fingers up again as I say the syllables: "ear" (*first finger up*) "ring" (*second finger up*). There are two syllables in the word 'earring.' Now what would be left if we took away 'ring' (*put second finger down*)? Just the syllable 'ear' would be left."
- "Get ready to put up your fingers as I say another word: 'book' (*put first finger up*) 'mark' (*put second finger up*). There are two syllables in that word too. Now let's take away 'book' (*put first finger down*). What syllable is left?"
- "Let's do one more before we read a book. 'Bas' (*put first finger up*) 'ket' (*put up second finger*) 'ball' (*put up third finger*). There are three syllables in the word basketball. What happens if we take away 'ball' (*put down third finger*). What two syllables are left in that word?"

Literature

Read *The Very Hungry Caterpillar* by Eric Carle.

- Count the number of syllables in words in the title by putting up fingers as you say the syllables in the words: *The* (1), *Very* (2), *Hungry* (2), *Caterpillar* (4).
- Count the number of syllables in some of the multisyllabic words in the book (e.g., Tuesday, salami, lollipop, cupcake, watermelon, hungry, cocoon, butterfly).
- After counting the number of syllables in a couple of the above words, ask the children what word would be left if you took one of the syllables away. For example, "cupcake" has two syllables. What would be left if you took away "cake"? (cup)

Whole-Class Activity

Preparation

- Copy and cut apart word cards.
- A puppet is also needed.

Activity

The teacher introduces the activity to the class.

- "Today we have a very hungry puppet with us. He is just like the very hungry caterpillar in the book we just read. Who can remember some of the kinds of food the caterpillar in the book ate? Well, this puppet is kind of funny—instead of eating food, he eats parts of words.

Your job is going to be to tell me what part of the word is left after he eats another part of the word."

- "We have some long words here. These words are written in a funny way so that one syllable is on each card. This puppet just eats one syllable out of the words and leaves the rest of the word behind. That's kind of like when the caterpillar in the book ate a hole in the food but left the rest of the food behind. Our puppet is looking awfully hungry, so we had better get some words out quickly to feed him."

Ask two children to come up to the front of the room. Give them each a card with one syllable of the word.

- Have the puppet read the word as he moves from the first child to the second child: "Mmmm, pop—corn. I'm going to eat the syllable 'pop.'" (Have the puppet put the card with "pop" written on it in his mouth.)
- Teacher: "We had the word 'popcorn' but now we can't say 'pop' because it's gone. What's left?" (Have the child who is holding the "corn" card tell you the answer.)

Ask three new children to come up to the front as the first two children sit down. Hand out strawberry syllable cards.

- Have the puppet read the word. The puppet decides to eat "straw."
- "Now we have the word 'strawberry,' but we can't say 'straw' because the puppet ate it. What is left in the word 'strawberry' without 'straw'?" (Two children holding "ber" and "ry" should say the names of their remaining pieces.)
- Continue the same pattern of activities for the following words:

  1. (2 syllables) cowboy (eat "boy")
  2. (3) waterslide (eat "slide")
  3. (2) coughdrop (eat "cough")
  4. (2) playground (eat "ground")
  5. (2) birthday (eat "day")
  6. (3) lawnmower (eat "lawn")
  7. (2) cupcake (eat "cake")
  8. (2) doorbell (eat "door")
  9. (3) cheeseburger (eat "cheese")
  10. (2) railroad (eat "road")
  11. (2) toothbrush (eat "tooth")
  12. (3) ladybug (eat "bug")
  13. (2) pancake (eat "pan")

Small-Group Activity

Preparation

- Copy and cut out caterpillar parts and put them in the center of the small-group table.
- Copy and cut up word cards for the small group. Keep the word cards by the teacher.

Activity

- Tell the children that they are going to listen to words and put one syllable of the word on each part of the caterpillar.
- Say the word "meatball." Have the children say it after you, putting one finger up for each syllable. Next, put the syllable card "meat" on the head of the caterpillar and the syllable "ball" on the middle body of the caterpillar; take away the tail end of the caterpillar because there are only two syllables in the word. Say the word "meatball" again as you point first to the head and then the body of the caterpillar. Now the caterpillar head is disconnected from the body, and the head with "meat" gets lost. Ask a child, "Now what's left of the word 'meatball' without the syllable 'meat'?" (Point to the body of the caterpillar.) Put the caterpillar parts back in the center. Do the next words in a similar manner.

  1. (3) dishwasher, lose "dish"
  2. (3) microwave, lose "wave"
  3. (2) eyebrow, lose "brow"
  4. (2) airplane, lose "air"
  5. (2) fireplace, lose "place"
  6. (2) scarecrow, lose "crow"
  7. (2) dollhouse, lose "doll"
  8. (3) grasshopper, lose "grass"

- If children are getting good at this task, you can make it harder by losing other syllables (e.g., lose "er" in "grasshopper"; "grasshopp" is left).
- You can also use cards from the whole-class activity and place them on the caterpillar or get the puppet out to use with the small group also.

Optional Related Activities

- During calendar time, ask children to say the names of days of the week or the names of months of the year without one of the syllables (e.g., "Say Friday; now say it again but don't say 'day'"; or "Say October; now say it again but don't say 'Oc'").

Materials Needed

Reproducible materials accompanying the lesson:

- Syllable word cards for the whole-class activity.
- Syllable word cards for the small-group activity.
- Caterpillar pieces picture for the small-group activity.

Other materials:

- Book: *The Very Hungry Caterpillar* by Eric Carle. New York: Philomel Books, 1987. ISBN: 0-399-20853-4.
- Puppet for the whole-class activity

Whole-Class Two-Syllable Word Cards (Lesson 7)

pop	corn
cow	boy
cough	drop
play	ground
birth	day
cup	cake
door	bell
rail	road
tooth	brush
pan	cake

Whole-Class Three-Syllable Word Cards (Lesson 7)

straw	ber	ry
wa	ter	slide
lawn	mow	er
cheese	bur	ger
la	dy	bug

Small-Group Syllable Word Cards (Lesson 7)

meat	ball
eye	brow
air	plane
scare	crow
doll	house

dish	wash	er
mi	cro	wave
com	put	er
grass	hopp	er

Caterpillar Picture for Small-Group Activity (Lesson 7)

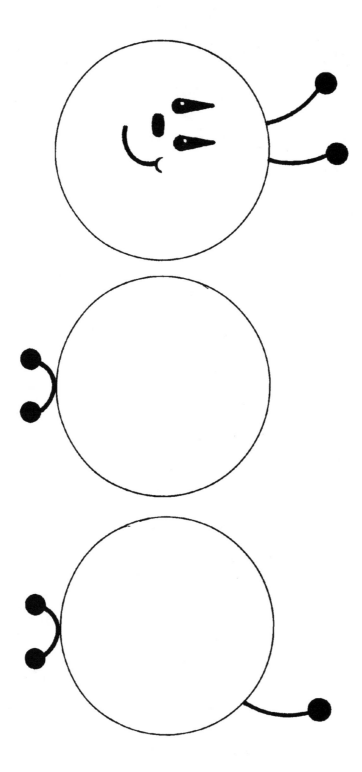

Lesson 8: Onset–Rime Blending

Introduction

Preparation

- Copy and cut apart introduction cards.
- Gather clothing items (sock, shoe, coat, hat, shorts, pants, shirt).

Activity

Hold up two pieces of the fish introduction cards, one in each hand, each containing an "onset" or a "rime" of the word.

- Tell the children that you are going to say the first sound of the word (the onset) and then the last part of the word (the rime). Tell them to try to guess the word.
- Say the onset sound. In the present case of "fish," for example, "The first sound is /fffff/."
- Say the sounds of the rime: "This is the end of the word; it says /ish/."
- Ask if any of the children know what the word is.
- Keep repeating the onset /f/ and the rime /ish/ with pauses in between while moving hands/cards together until finally they are right next to each other; then say the word.
- Do another example for the class and model for the class saying the onset /s/ and rime /un/ with a shorter and shorter pause between them until it is easy to figure out what the word is: "sun."

Place clothing out on a table for the class to choose from. Words/items: s—ock, sh—oe, c—oat, h—at, sh—orts, p—ants, sh—irt.

- Name all of the items of clothing before you begin the activity.
- Explain to the children that you are going to say the names of those items but you're going to say them in a funny way. You are going to say the beginning sound of the word separated from the rest of the word. Tell them that they will need to listen very carefully so that they can put the sounds together and can then guess which word you said.
- Say the name of one of the items with the first sound segmented from rest of word (e.g., "sh—orts"). Have the children guess which of the items you said. Continue with each of the other items, with children guessing after each which word you said.

Practice the skill without a set of objects to choose from.

- Tell children that you will say the names of some other items in the room and they have to guess what you've said.
- Here are some examples of items in the room you might name:

  1. d—oor
  2. ch—alk

3. d—esk
4. ch—air

Literature

Read *There's a Bug in My Mug* by Kent Salisbury.

- Point out the rhyming words in the book to the children as you read.
- Show the children how as the picture changes from one rhyming word to another, the end of the rhyming word stays the same and just the first letter/sound changes to make the different word.
- For example, on the first page of the book, point out that the word "mug" starts with the /m/ sound. The letter "m" is written in pink in the book. When the arrow is pushed in the book so that the picture changes from mug to bug, a green letter "b" covers the "m" and now the word is "bug."

Whole-Class Activity

"Simon Says" Activity

- Tell the children that the class is going to play a game called "Simon Says": "The object of the game is to listen carefully and do *only* what Simon tells you to do. If Simon doesn't tell you to do something, don't move."
- "When I'm telling you what Simon says to do, I'm going to say some of the words slowly in pieces. You need to listen carefully so you can figure out what Simon wants you to do."

    1. Simon says touch your n—ose.
    2. Simon says shake your f—oot.
    3. Look at the d—oor.
    4. Simon says touch your l—eg.
    5. Simon says put your hands on your h—ead.
    6. S—it down.
    7. Simon says look at the w—all.
    8. Simon says st—and.
    9. Move your h—and.
    10. Simon says touch your kn—ee.
    11. Simon says j—ump.

Small-Group Activity

Preparation

- Copy and cut apart small-group picture cards.
- Put pictures from a different rhyme family in front of each child (one child with pictures that end with "ug" sounds, another child with pictures that end with "ow" sounds, etc.).

Activity

- Say the name of one of the pictures (in front of one of the children) with the onset separated from the rime.
- Ask whose set of pictures the word you said is in.
- After the right child answers, have him or her listen as you say the rime portion and some of the words in the group he or she chose to confirm or deny the answer: "Do you hear /ug/ in 'rug,' 'mug,' and 'bug'? Yes, you are correct." Or "Do you hear /ug/ in 'bow,' 'mow,' 'snow'? No, you're right. You don't hear /ug/ in the ends of those words."
- Say the word again with the onset separated from the rime and ask the child to choose which picture you said.
- The task can be made more difficult as the children's proficiency improves by mixing pictures from rhyme families together on the table.
- The task can be made even more difficult by removing picture choices totally. Children must then rely on auditory/visual information from the teacher's production of the onset separated from the rime to blend onset–rime to guess the word.

Optional Related Activities

- Make paper turkeys during an art activity with different onsets/initial sounds on each feather and rime on the turkey body.
- Buy plastic or other disposable gloves. Write onset on fingers of the glove and rime on the palm of the glove.
- Read other "pop into phonics" books such as *A Bear Ate My Pear* (by Kent Saisbury. New York: McClanahan, 1998. ISBN: 0-76-810026-7) or *My Nose Is a Hose* (by Kent Saisbury. New York: McClanahan, 1997. ISBN: 1-56-293930-0.

Materials Needed

Reproducible materials accompanying the lesson:

- Introduction word cards (fish, sun).
- Rhyme group pictures for the small group.

Other materials:

- Book: *There's a Bug in My Mug* by Kent Saisbury. New York: McClanahan, 1997. ISBN: 1-56293-931-9.
- Clothing items for introduction choices: socks, shoes, coat, hat, shorts, pants, shirt.

Introduction Cards (Lesson 8)

f | ish

s | un

Small-Group Pictures (Lesson 8)

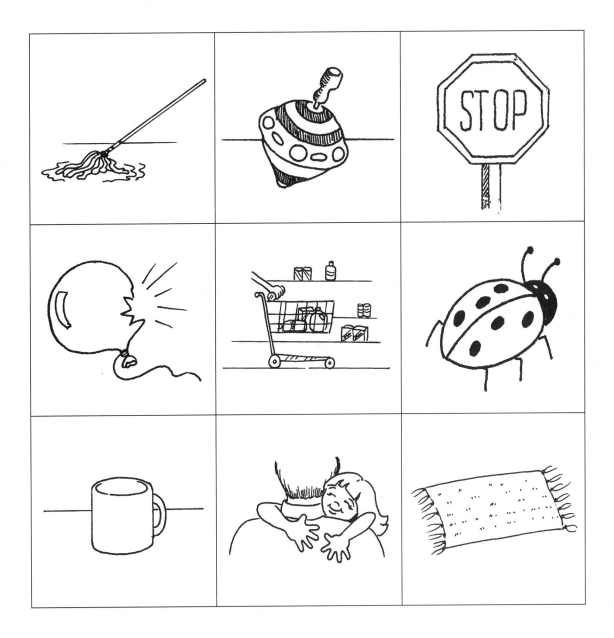

Small-Group Pictures (Lesson 8)

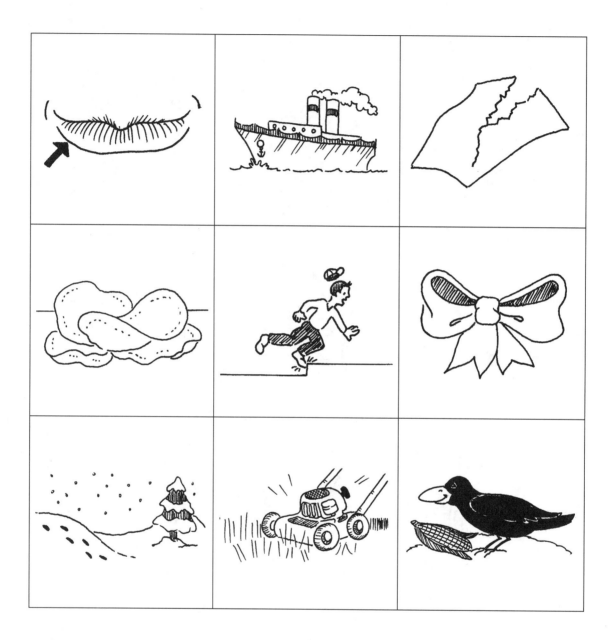

Small-Group Pictures (Lesson 8)

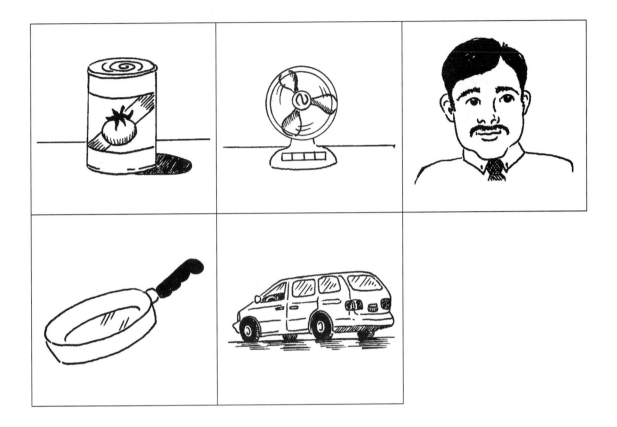

Lesson 9: Onset–Rime Blending

Introduction

Preparation

- Copy and cut apart onset–rime clue cards.
- Put each mystery picture in a different envelope.
- *Optional*: Dress up like a private detective (with a hat and trench coat).

Activity

Optional: Ask children who they think you're pretending to be. Explain that you are dressed like a detective who sometimes looks for clues:

- "Today we are going to hear a detective story and pretend to be detectives."
- "Last week we were listening to words that had the beginning sound separated from the rest of the word. We put the first sound together with the rest of the word to figure out the word. Today we are going to pretend those parts of the words are clues, and our job is to listen to the clues and figure out what the mystery picture is in the envelopes."
- First Mystery (clues: r—ed, fr—uit; picture in envelop 1: apple):

  1. "Here's our first clue." Hold up two pieces of paper, one in each hand, containing an onset and a rime that make up a word. Say the sound of the onset, /r/. Then say the sound of the rime, /ed/. Keep repeating the onset and the rime with shorter and shorter pauses between them while moving your hands slowly closer together until finally they are right next to each other; then say the clue word. Continue: "Here's our next clue" (fr—uit). Call on the class to decide what the next clue is. After the class figures out the word "fruit," ask: "What do you think the clues are describing? What's a red fruit? Let's look in the First Mystery envelope and see if you're right."
  2. Repeat with the Second Mystery (clues: b—ig, c—at, r—oar; picture in envelope 2: lion).
  3. Repeat with the Third Mystery (clues: f—arm, e—gg, cl—uck; picture in envelope 3: chicken).

Literature

- Read *The ABC Mystery* by Doug Cushman.
- Possible unfamiliar words that may require explanation throughout the above book:

  1. A—art—A picture that was hanging on the wall.
  2. B—butler—Someone who works at people's houses and answers the door.
  3. C—clue—The flower laying on the ground was in the butler's coat. It might give the police a hint of who took the picture.
  4. D—detective—A kind of policeman whose job is to solve mysteries.

5. I—inspector—Another word that means detective, often a policeman of higher rank.
6. J—jalopy—An old car.
7. K—kilt—A knee-length pleated skirt often worn by Scotsmen, including Scottish soldiers.
8. M—manor—A big house in the country.
9. Q—query—A question; also, to ask a question.
10. R—robber—Someone who steals things from others.
11. T—tunnel—A long underground passageway.
12. V—vault—A safe place in which to keep valuable things.
13. W—wombat—An Australian animal resembling a small bear.

- Discuss events or terms from the book while practicing onset–rime blending. For example: "In the story the detective drove a jalopy. A jalopy is an old c—ar. The detective drove to a manor looking for the stolen painting. A manor is a big h—ouse in the country."

Whole-Class Activity

Preparation for the Scavenger Hunt

- Look for one-syllable objects/places around your room. Write the first sound or sound cluster (onset) on front of an index card; write the rime portion of the word on back of the same index card.
- Ideas of single syllable objects/places that may be in your room that could be used as clues include: fl-ag, d-oor, ph-one, b-ooks, t-ape, ch-alk, ch-air, d-esk, b-ox, sh-elf.
- You can include an extra clue on the card to help narrow down where the next card is hidden after the mystery word on the card is guessed. For example, after "desk" is guessed by the class, you can note that another clue on the card says "teacher," so the next clue must be near the teacher's desk. Another clue might be the color of a particular chair in the room, where the next clue is hidden, and so on.
- Arrange index clue cards around the room for the hunt. You keep the first clue with you. For example, the card you keep might say "fl-ag"; under the flag you put a card that says "d-oor"; at the door you place a card that says "b-ox"; under a box in your room you place the card that says "ch-alk." At the last place in the scavenger hunt the last clue directs the children to a place where some kind of treasure (e.g., a snack, stickers) is hidden.

Scavenger Hunt

- Explain to the children that now they get to be detectives too. "There are clues with mystery words hidden around the room. We have to follow the clues and guess the mystery words to find a treasure at the end of our hunt."
- Orchestrate scavenger hunt(s). A small group of children can help you look for the next clue. Everyone in the class, or just the children who helped find the clue, can guess the mystery word as you say the clue word's onset separated by a pause from the word's rime. Have the first group of children sit down and choose another small group of children to find the next card, and so on.

Small-Group Activity

Preparation

- Copy and cut apart onset–rime small-group cards.
- Mix and place small-group cards face down on the table in rows and columns for a memory game.

Activity

Play the "Mystery Memory" game.

- Children take turns turning over two cards.
- If the two cards have the same symbols on them, the children have a match that forms a mystery word.
- If the symbols don't match, the children turn the cards back over and it is the next child's turn.
- When they get a match, the teacher may ask what sound the onset letter makes. The teacher then says the onset sound with a brief pause, followed by the rime portion of the word.
- If a child is having difficulty guessing the word, have him or her repeat saying onset–rime portions after you. Lengthen the onset sound as you say it if it is a continuous sound (/f/, /v/, /h/, /m/, /n/, /s/, /v/, /ʃ/ [*sh*]), and decrease the pause time between onset and rime.
- Repeat the game as time allows.

Optional Related Activities

- Play the "I Spy" game. The teacher looks around the room and says, "I spy something. It's a c—oat." You can give additional clues: "I spy something Jenny's wearing. It's a r—ing." Or "I spy something that rings. It's a b—ell." You can also do "I'm thinking of something that . . . " so that the game is not limited just to objects in your room.

Materials Needed

Reproducible materials accompanying the lesson:

- Onset–rime clue cards and mystery pictures for the introduction.
- Onset–rime cards for the small-group matching game.

Other materials:

- Book: *The ABC Mystery* by Doug Cushman. New York: HarperCollins, 1993. ISBN: 0-06-021227-6.
- A trench coat, a magnifying glass, and a hat so the teacher can dress up as a private detective during the introduction and whole-class activity.
- Three envelopes to put three mystery pictures in for the introduction.
- Index cards with one-syllable words written on them of items in the classroom for the whole-class scavenger hunt.
- Prize (stickers or a snack, etc.) to be found at end of the scavenger hunt.

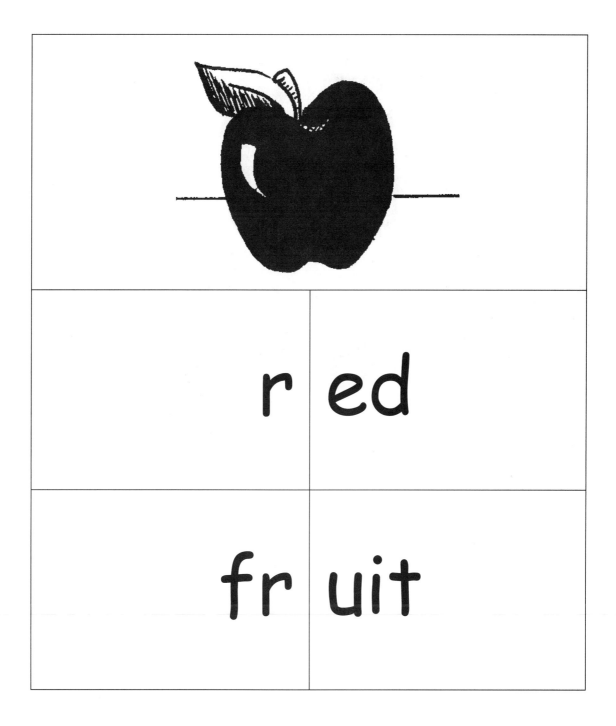

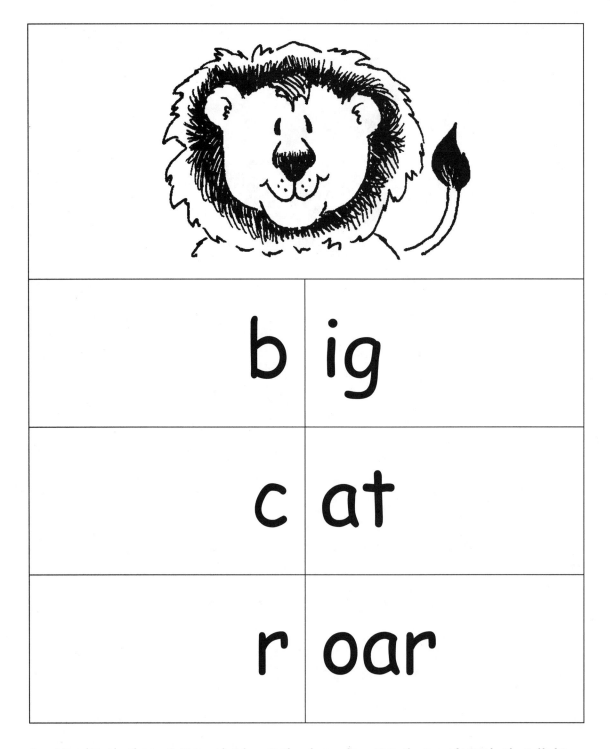

b	ig
c	at
r	oar

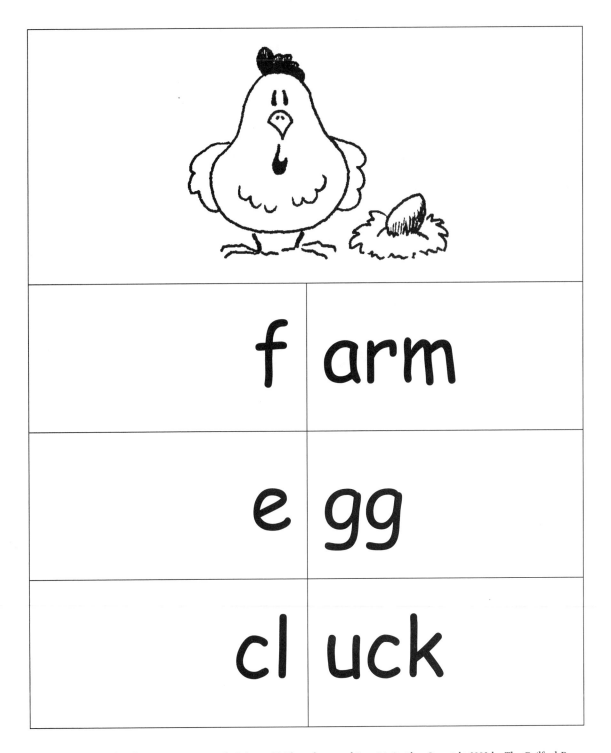

Small-Group Onset–Rime Matching Cards (Lesson 9)

♥ m	♥ om	☺ f	☺ eet
♦ h	♦ ot	♣ n	♣ ap
✔ l	✔ eg	☼ f	☼ un
✉ b	✉ all	❽ s	❽ it
♦ n	♦ ail	📖 d	📖 og
☞ g	☞ oat	☎ h	☎ and
✎ j	✎ ump	✈ k	✈ ite
🕐 l	🕐 amb	☆ m	☆ ilk
❄ s	❄ oap	♣ t	♣ ape

Lesson 10: Review of Rhyming and of Syllable and Onset–Rime Blending

Introduction

Explain that the class has learned so many things about words and that "today we are going to combine them all together to see how much we know."

- "Today we are going to do three different things. First we are going to listen to big pieces of words or syllables and blend them together to figure out what word is being said. Let's do a few practice words. Listen closely to the syllables and raise your hand if you know what word I said"
- cow—boy
- play—ground
- wa—ter—fall
- tel—e—phone

"We are also going to think about rhyming words today. Remember words that rhyme sound the same at the ends of the words but have different beginning sounds. Do these words rhyme?"

- ring–sun (No, they don't rhyme; "ing–un," ends of words, are different.)
- ring–sing (Yes, they rhyme; both words end with "ing.")
- ring–red (No, they don't rhyme; the ends of the words are different, "ing–ed.")

"Now let's think of some words that rhyme. Tell me a real or silly word that rhymes with . . . "

- bed
- hot
- cow

"Now listen carefully and tell me what word I'm saying. Listen to the first sound and the rest of the word; then put the pieces together to figure out what word I'm saying."

- f—an
- p—ig
- m—ilk
- j—ump

Whole-Class Activity 1

Preparation

- Copy the Class Activity 1 page for each child in the class.
- Each child needs a pencil (or another writing instrument) for the task.

Activity

"Everyone will need a pencil out. Let's look at the pictures on your paper. There is a dinosaur, a grasshopper, a hamburger, cereal, a caterpillar, and a calendar. We are going to draw lines connecting some of the pictures. Listen carefully and do draw the lines. Please don't talk or say the answers during this lesson."

- "Put your pencil on the calendar at the bottom of the page. Draw a line to the ca—ter—pil—lar."
- "Now put your pencil on the dinosaur. Draw a line to the grass—hop—per."
- "Put your pencil on the hamburger. Draw a line to the di—no—saur."
- "Put your pencil on the hamburger again. Draw a line to the ce—re—al."
- "Put your pencil on the caterpillar. Draw a line to the ham–bur—ger."

The teacher can view accuracy quickly looking at the page. The lines will look like a capital **E** if all of the items are correct. Have each child put his or her name on the page and give the page to you so that accuracy for each can be analyzed.

Whole-Class Activity 2

"We are going to play 'Simon Says' with rhyming words and listening for syllables in words. Everyone stand up and get in a circle. Listen carefully and do *only* what Simon tells you to do. Otherwise, do nothing."

- Simon says touch the part of you face that rhymes with "hose." (nose)
- Simon says look at the cal—en—der.
- Simon says start jump—ing.
- Simon says stop jump—ing.
- Simon says rub your tummy if you like to eat ba—na—nas.
- Touch your shoul—der.
- Simon says look at a com—put—er.
- Simon says touch the part of your head that rhymes with "fear." (ear)

Whole-Class Activity 3

Preparation

- Copy the Class Activity 3 page for each child in the class.
- Each child needs a pencil (or another writing instrument) for the task.

Activity

"Everyone will need a pencil out. Let's look at the pictures on your paper. They show feet, rain, a rip, a fan, and a ship. We are going to draw lines connecting some of the pictures. Listen carefully and draw the lines. Please don't talk or say the answers during this lesson."

- Put your pencil at the bottom of the page on the fan. Draw a line to the f—eet.
- Put your pencil on the rip. Draw a line to the r—ain.
- Put your pencil on the feet. Draw a line to the sh—ip.
- Put your pencil on the ship. Draw a line to the r—ain.
- Put your pencil on the rip. Draw a line to the f—an.

The teacher can check accuracy quickly by viewing each child's page. The lines will look like a five-pointed star if all of the items are correct.

Materials Needed

Reproducible materials accompanying the lesson:

- One copy of the Whole-Class Lesson Activity 1 page for each child in the class.
- One copy of the Whole-Class Lesson Activity 3 page for each child in the class.

Other materials:

- Each child needs a pencil or another writing instrument.

Whole-Class Activity 1 (Lesson 10)

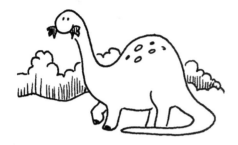

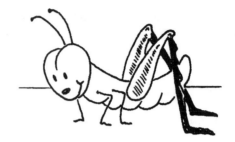

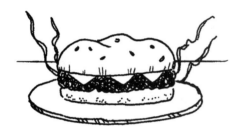

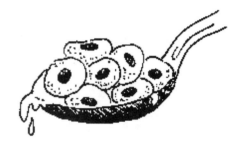

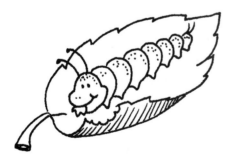

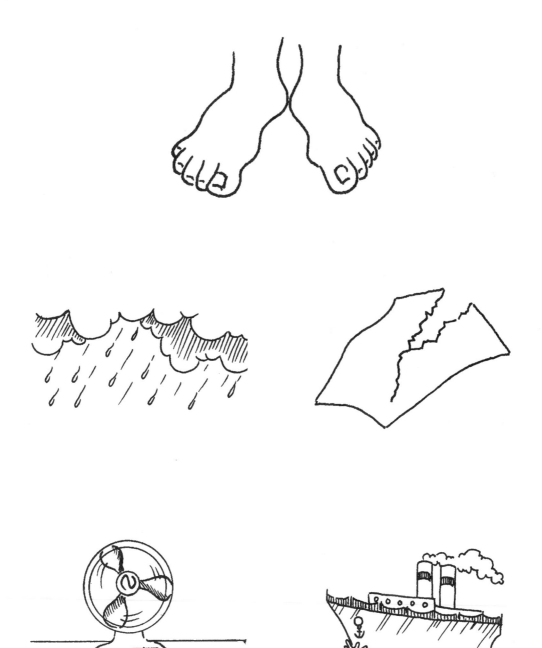

Lesson 11: Initial Phoneme Identification

Introduction

Explain the concept of identifying the first sound in a word:

- "Who can tell me what the very first sound in their name is?" Use the example to further explain the concept to the class. For example, if the child's name was Sam, say "Yes, Sam, the first sound in your name is /sss/." If the child responded with the letter name, say "The first letter in your name is *s*, but the first sound is /sss/. Your name also has the sounds /a/ and /mmm/, but the first sound is /sss/."
- Have the class stand up. Tell the children to sit down if their name starts with the sound you say. Proceed to say the first sound of some of the children's names until all the children are sitting down. For example, "If your name starts with /fff/, sit down. If your name starts with /t/, sit down." If a child—say, Tim—does not sit down when he is supposed to, prompt him by saying, "Tim, what is the first sound in your name?"

Literature

Read *What Am I?: An Animal Guessing Game* by Iza Trapani.

- Each time the children guess an animal in the book or the page has been turned to reveal the animal, discuss the first sound of the animal's name. For example, "Yes, the animal that claps his flippers is a sssseal. The first sound in sssseal is /sss/."

Whole-Class Activity

Preparation

- Copy and cut apart the animal pictures included for the whole-class activity. Tape the pictures onto a large ball (face down so the children cannot see the pictures).

Activity

- Gently roll the ball across the circle to a child. Have that child roll the ball back to you. Take a picture off the ball and give the child clues about the pictured animal (similar to the story). For example, if the picture was a whale, you might say, "This is a type of animal that lives in the ocean. It is big and squirts water out of its head." Once the child guesses whale, ask the child what the first sound in the word is.
- If the child has difficulty guessing the sound, exaggerate the production of /w/ by puckering your lips and prolonging the sound a little. Say, "The first sound in 'whale' is . . . (*pucker your lips but slow down enunciation of the sound*)."
- Proceed around the circle until all the children have a turn.

Small-Group Activity

Preparation

- Copy bingo cards. Markers on the bingo card (e.g., chips, tokens) are also needed.

Activity

- Provide each child with a bingo card. Explain to the children that they need to place chips or tokens on the pictures of the bingo cards when they have identified a picture that begins with a certain sound. Then say a sound (listed below) and the children will need to find one picture on the card that has that sound at the beginning of its name. The children will cover up the picture on the card with a token or chip. Bingo is achieved when the chips on the pictures are in a row across, down, or diagonally. Once a child has bingo, he or she yells it out, switches cards, and plays another game.
- Use the following sounds for the pictured items: /p/, /b/, /d/, /f/, /h/, /j/, /m/, /n/, /r/, /t/, /w/, /v/, /k/, /g/, /l/, and /s/.
- If a child has difficulty, point to a picture on the card and say the word emphasizing the first sound. Ask if the child hears the target sound at the beginning. If he or she does not, point to a picture that does have the target sound, look at the child, and say the sound clearly. Ask the child if he or she has now heard the target sound.

Optional Related Activities

- Provide the children with a sound. Have a child go around the room and find something that begins with that sound. For example, "Children, the sound is /fff/. Jason, can you find something in the room that begins with /fff/?" Jason points to the number 5 on the number strip in the classroom.
- Consider an alternative to this activity and have the children describe the item they have found that begins with a certain sound. See if the other children can guess what the object is.

Materials Needed

Reproducible materials accompanying the lesson:

- Pictures of animals to place on the ball.
- Bingo cards.

Other materials:

- Book, *What Am I?: An Animal Guessing Game* by Iza Trapani. Boston: Whispering Coyote Press, 1992. ISBN: 1-879085-66-6.
- Ball for the whole-class activity.
- Tape for the whole-class activity.
- Chips or tokens for bingo for the small-group activity.

Pictures for Whole-Class Activity (Lesson 11)

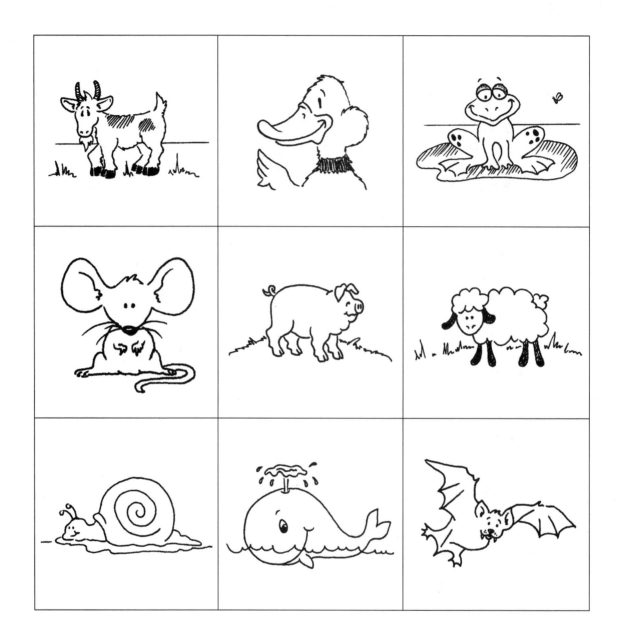

Pictures for Whole-Class Activity (Lesson 11)

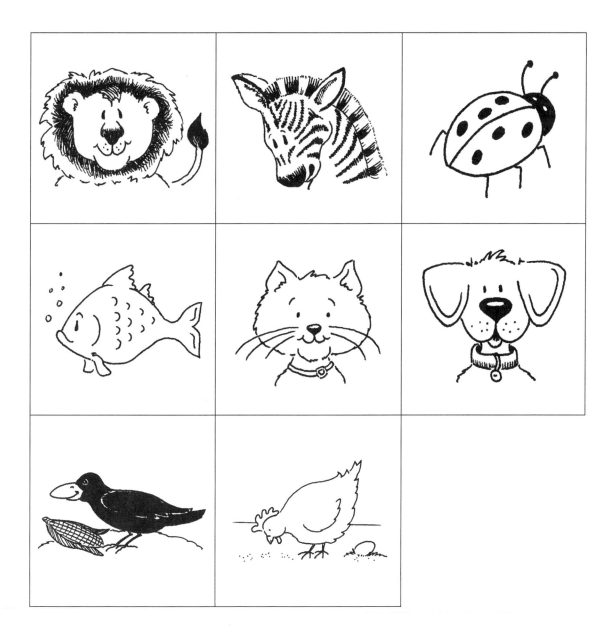

Small-Group Bingo Cards (Lesson 11)

BINGO

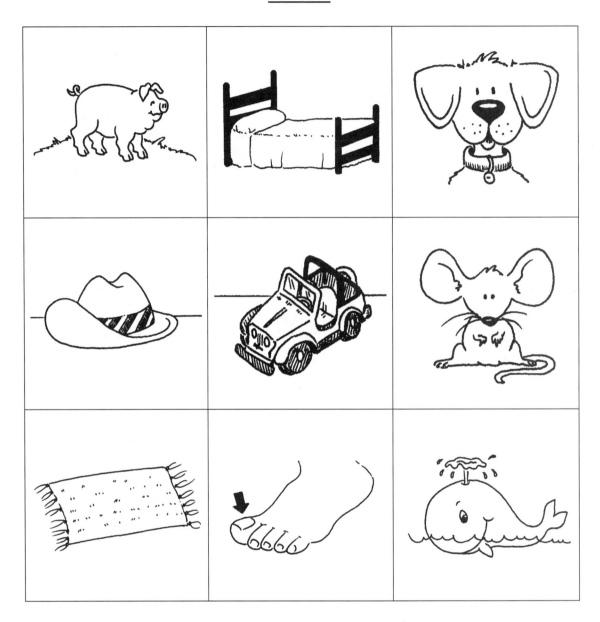

Small-Group Bingo Cards (Lesson 11)

BINGO

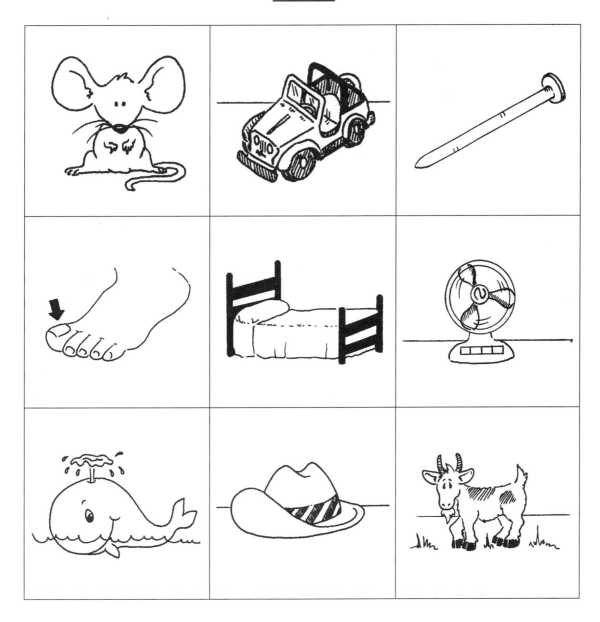

Small-Group Bingo Cards (Lesson 11)

BINGO

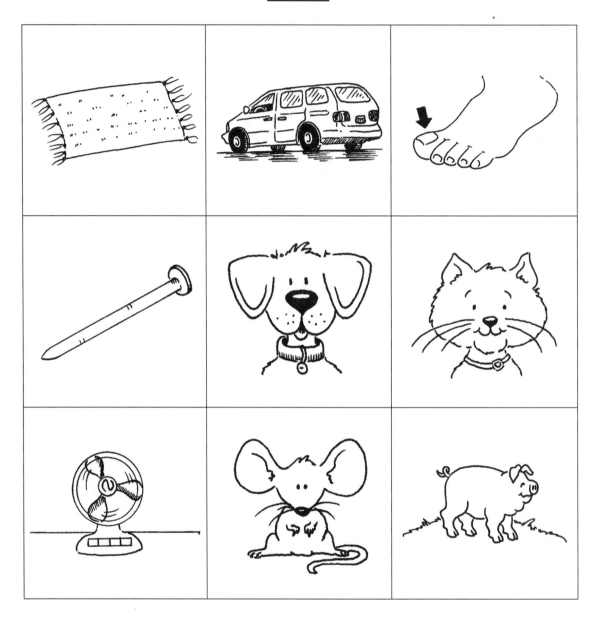

Small-Group Bingo Cards (Lesson 11)

BINGO

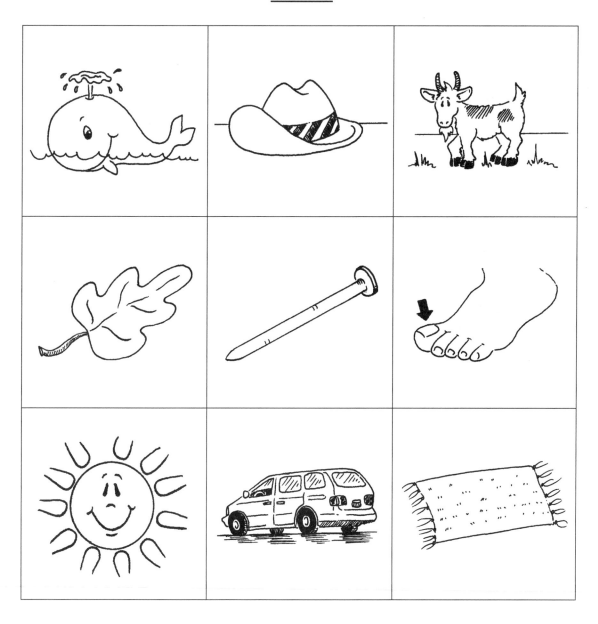

Small-Group Bingo Cards (Lesson 11)

$\underline{BINGO}$

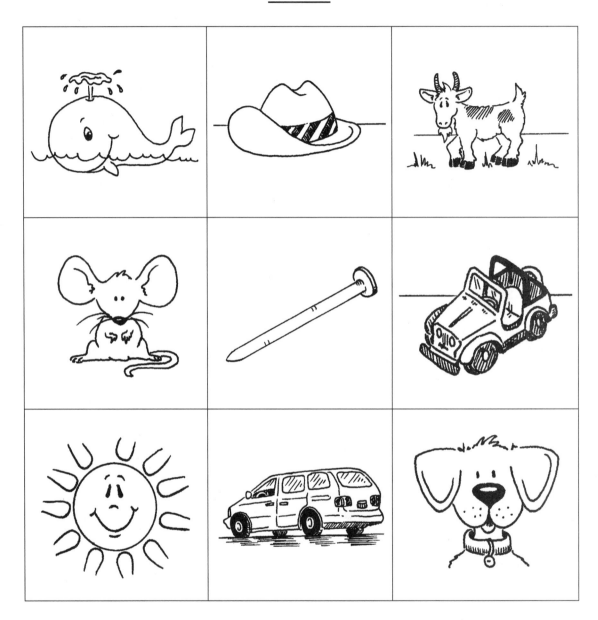

Lesson 12: Initial Phoneme Production

Introduction

Review the concept of beginning sounds in words:

- "Today, we are going to listen to the beginnings of words. For example, when I say the word 'soup,' the first sound in that word is /sssss/, the middle sound is /oooo/, and the last sound is /p/.
- "What is the first sound in the word 'four'?"

Involve the children in a guessing game to see who can guess the first sound in words (e.g., zebra, horse, deer, lizard, spider, cheetah, parrot, etc.).

- "We are going to play a guessing game today to see who can listen and say the beginning sounds in words."
- Ask a child to come to the front of the class and think of a word to say aloud. Let the child say the word and have the classmates raise their hand if they think they know the first sound in the word.
- Continue with a few children providing appropriate feedback to the responses. Provide additional information when needed. For example, the child says "fish," and the classmate guesses the first sound as /ʃ/ (*sh*). Say, "That's a good guess because /ʃ/ is in the word, but let's listen to the very beginning of the word 'ffffish.' What sound was at the beginning?").

Literature

Read *Kids Celebrate the Alphabet* by Teresa Walsh.

- Stop periodically throughout the book and ask the children to listen for the sound at the beginning of the words you say.
- For example, one of the verses in the book is "*D* is for dinosaur, doctor, and doll. *D* is for dog, who comes when I call." Say, "Children, the letter is *d*, the sound is /d/ (*make the sound*). Listen to these two words and tell me which word has the /d/ sound in it, call or dog. That's right, dog has the /d/ sound at the beginning of the word. Call has the /k/ sound."
- Ask the children what sound certain words start with; for example, "What sound does goat begin with?" If they guess the sound, ask for another word that starts with that same sound.

Whole-Class Activity

Preparation

- A puppet is needed.

Activity

- The teacher says a sound, the puppet says a word, and the class has to judge whether the word started with the sound the teacher said or not.
- For example, the teacher says the /l/ sound and the puppet says "hat." The teacher responds: "Children, does hat begin with the /l/ sound?" A few more examples might be provided (e.g., teacher says /p/, puppet says pie; teacher says /f/, puppet says finger; teacher says /g/, puppet says water).
- For another activity, have a child come forward. Explain that a puppet will say a sound and the child needs to think of a word that begins with the sound the puppet said. If the child says a word that does not begin with the sound, ask the class if they can think of a word that does begin with that sound.
- For a third activity, walk around the class and give the puppet to children who have not had a turn previously. The teacher says a word to the child with the puppet, and the child then has the puppet tell the class the beginning sound in the word.

Small-Group Activity

Preparation

- Put objects in a paper bag (pencil, pen, paper, rock, ring, raisin, dime, duck, doll, tape, tack, tie). Another option is to put other objects you would like to use in a bag and write them down so you can provide the initial sounds.

Activity

- Explain to the children that they are going to try to find something in the bag that starts with the sound you give them.
- Give the children one of the four sounds being targeted: /p/, /r/, /d/, or /t/. For example, "Children, the first sound is /p/. Let's see who can find something in the bag that begins with the /p/ sound. When the child draws an object, ask if the object begins with /p/. If it does, keep the object out of the bag. If the child chooses an object that does not begin with /p/, have them tell you the beginning sound of the object they drew. Proceed until all objects are out of the bag.

Optional Related Activities

Further explain the concept of beginning, middle, and end in concrete ways:

- As children line up at the door, ask the class who is at the beginning of the line and who is at the end, and have all the others in the middle raise their hands.
- Use this concept to explain a word. "If the line was the word 'bat,' Susie in front would be /b/, all of you in the middle would be /a/, and John at the end would be /t/. The beginning sound of the word is /b/, the middle is /a/, and the end is /t/."

Materials Needed

No reproducible materials needed.

Other materials:

- Book: *Kids Celebrate the Alphabet* by Teresa Walsh. Everett, WA: Warren, 1996. ISBN: 1-57029-162-4.
- A puppet for the whole-class activity.
- A brown paper bag for the small-group activity.
- Objects to put in the bag (pencil, pen, paper, rock, ring, raisin, dime, duck, doll, tape, tack, tie) for the small-group activity.

Lesson 13: Final Phoneme Identification

Introduction

Preparation

- Copy the drawing of a train provided with this lesson.

Activity

Discuss sounds at the end of words.

- Use the train provided to point out to the children the beginning of the train, the middle, and the end. "The beginning of the train is the engine, the middle is a train car, and the end of the train is a caboose." Compare a train to a word. Some words have a beginning, middle, and end. For example, the word "pig" has a beginning/engine sound /p/, a middle sound /i/, and an end/caboose sound /g/.
- "We are going to use the train to help us remember that today we are listening for the last sound in words or the caboose sound."
- Say the word "mad." Ask the children if they can figure out what the last sound in the word is. When they say /d/, say "Yes, the last sound is /d/." While pointing at the train, say "The first sound is /m/, the middle sound is /a/, and the last sound is /d/." Give other examples of consonant-vowel-consonant words (cut, pan, mop, sit, etc.).

Literature

Read *The Caboose Who Got Loose* by Bill Peet.

- Emphasize the caboose is at the end of the train just like the sounds we are listening for today.
- Periodically ask the children what sound is at the end of certain words in the story.

Whole-Class Activity

The whole-class activity will involve children guessing which child in front of the classroom is the caboose sound or last sound in a word.

- Tell the class the word they need to be thinking of is "dig." Tell them to be thinking about the end of the word, but they need to be quiet. One of their classmates will be the caboose sound, and they have to guess who it is.
- Have three children go to the back of the classroom. Give each child a sound to say. Ask them to whisper the sound to you. Put the children in a different order each time.
- Say to the class, "The train is ready to go. Remember, the word is 'dig' and you need to be thinking about the last sound in the word."

- Have the children chug to the front of the classroom by placing their hands on each other's waist. After they chug to the front of the classroom, ask them to say their sounds.
- See if the class can guess which child is the last sound or the caboose in the word "dig." If Jane is /i/, Doug is /g/, and Sue is /d/, then Doug is the caboose in the word dig. Once the class has figured out who the caboose sound is, put the children in order from left to right and model the word (Sue is first /d/, Jane is second /i/, and Doug is third /g/). Continue until each child has had a turn. Sample words to use include sack, big, chill, bed, fit, gum, ham, rat, ten, jet, luck, dip, win, pack, sad, dog, cut, run, mop, sit, fun, hid, pan, and need.

Small-Group Activity

Preparation

- Copy the train included in the reproducible material for each child in the small group.

Activity

- Tell the children they will be listening for the ending sounds in words and review the parts of a train with them and then review the beginning, middle, and end of a word.
- Tell the children a consonant-vowel-consonant word (e.g., log). Choose the words from the list provided for the whole class activity. Ask them to listen and concentrate on the end of the word. Have them point to the caboose of their train when they think they know the last sound in the word.
- Provide feedback such as "Yes, /d/ is the last sound in the word 'food'; /f/ is the engine or first sound (*point to the train*), /oo/ is the middle sound, and /d/ is the caboose or last sound."
- If children continue to struggle with final sounds, emphasize the beginning and middle sounds for them and let them fill in the last sound. For example, "The word is 'gum': /g/ is the first sound, /u/ is the second sound, and the last sound is ____." A contextual cue could also be used such as "I like to chew 'gu__.'"

Optional Related Activities

Talk about the final sounds in words throughout other activities during the day. For example, during calendar time, if the word sun comes up, ask someone if they know what the last sound or the caboose sound is in the word.

Materials Needed

Reproducible materials accompanying the lesson:

- Train for introduction and small group.

Other materials:

- Book: *The Caboose Who Got Loose* by Bill Peet. Boston: Houghton Mifflin, 1971. ISBN: 0-395-14805-7.

Drawing of a Train for the Introduction, Whole-Class, and Small-Group Activities (Lesson 13)

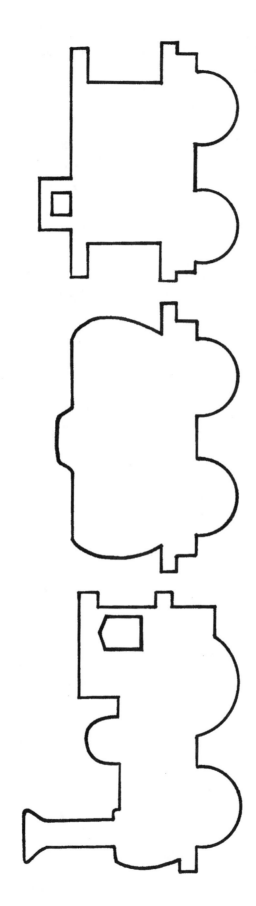

Lesson 14: Final Phoneme Production

Introduction

Preparation

- Gather three puppets; copy and cut apart the accompanying letter cards for use with the sounds if most of the class has an understanding of sound–symbol correspondences (see below).

Activity

Review the concept of final sounds in words.

- Have children guess what the final sound is in words presented to them (e.g., hug, sat, and five).
- Ask three children to come to the front of the classroom. Give each child a puppet, and whisper a sound from a consonant-vowel-consonant word to each child. Have the children make the puppet say the sound. Tell the class the word, and have the children decide which puppet has the last sound in the word. For example, whisper /a/ into one child's ear, /t/ into another, and /p/ into the last child's ear. Ask the three children whose puppet said the last sound in the word "tap." Once the answer is given, arrange the children and puppets in the correct order for their sounds and model the word to the class.
- If many children have an understanding of sound–symbol correspondence, consider using letter cards along with the sounds. Have the children hold the letter cards backwards so the class cannot see the letters. Each child should say the sound and then show the class his or her letter. The teacher should reinforce which child has the last sound in the word. The teacher says the word and asks the children to decide which child's letter makes the last sound in the word.
- Sample words that can be used for the introduction include pig, bad, fan, lap, mat, wet, hen, pet, hot, kid, bad, and dip.

Literature

Read *The Icky Sticky Anteater* by Dawn Bentley.

- Ask the child to identify the final sound in words of the book (e.g., job, hole, mole, lake, shout, sad, ant, night).
- Consider asking rhyming questions since many of the words rhyme in this book.

Whole-Class Activity

Preparation

- Copy and cut out picture cards included in this lesson. A container in which to place the pictures is also needed.

Activity

- Write five letters (i.e., *t, s, p, n, l*) on the chalkboard, and review the sounds with the children. Discuss how the class will be thinking about these sounds at the end of words during this activity.
- Put the pictures included with this lesson in a container. Have a child come forward, pick out a picture, and tell the class what the picture is. Ask the child, "What is the last sound in the word _____?" If the child responds correctly, place a little bit of sticky tack on the back of the picture and have the child place the picture under the correct letter on the chalkboard. If the child says the letter name, respond by saying, *t* is the letter; what is the sound?"

Small-Group Activity

Preparation

- The small-group activity consists of playing a memory game with the same cards used in the whole-class activity. Place 24 picture cards face down on the table.

Activity

- Explain to the children that they will be playing a different game of memory. The pictures will not match exactly, but they are to find two pictures with the same ending sound. If they find two pictures with the same ending sound, they get to keep the match.
- Have each child take a turn playing memory to see if the pictures have the same ending sound. As each picture is turned over, the child should name the picture and state the final sound in the word.
- If any children have difficulty with this, say the beginning of the word and leave off the final sound. Have the child say the final sound.
- After all the cards have been matched, have children name their matching pairs and identify the ending sound.
- If time allows, reshuffle the cards and repeat the activity.

Optional Related Activities

- Ask the children to bring back an item from home with a specified ending sound. Review the items with the whole class, emphasizing the specific sound at the end of the word.

Materials Needed

Reproducible materials accompanying the lesson:

- 24 pictures (4–5 pictures with the final sounds of /t/, /s/, /p/, /n/, and /l/) for the whole-class and small-group activities.
- Letter cards (if needed) for the introduction.

Other materials:

- Book: *The Icky Sticky Anteater* by Dawn Bentley. Santa Monica, CA: Piggy Toes Press, 2000. ISBN: 1-58117-121-8.
- Sticky tack for the whole-class activity.
- Puppets for the introduction.

Picture Cards for Whole-Class and Small-Group Activities (Lesson 14)
(Final Sounds /p/, /s/, /n/)

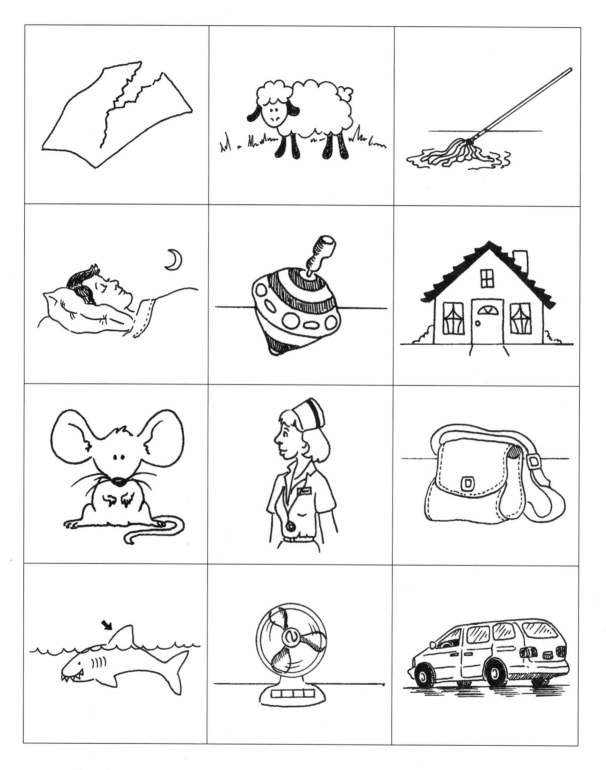

Picture Cards for Whole-Class and Small-Group Activities (Lesson 14)
(Final Sounds /n/, /l/, /t/)

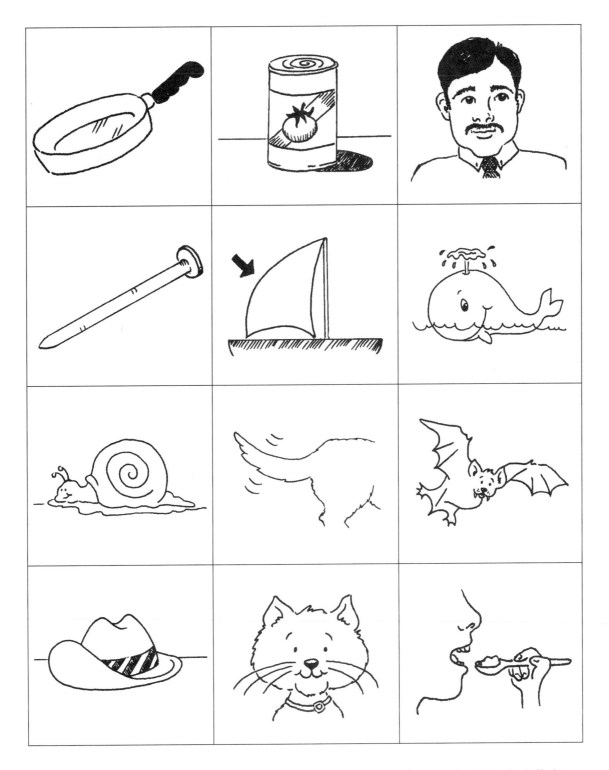

Letter Cards for Introduction (Lesson 14)

a	b	c	d
e	f	g	h
i	j	k	l
m	n	o	p
q	r	s	t
u	v	w	x
y	z		

Lesson 15: Medial Phoneme Isolation

Introduction

Preparation

- A puppet and paper Oreo-like cookies are needed materials.

Activity

Discuss sounds in the middle of words.

- Review with the children how the class has listened for beginning and ending sounds in words in the last few lessons: "Now, we are going to listen for the middle sounds."
- Talk about how many times the middle sounds in words are vowels. Vowels are sounds where our mouths are more open (e.g., /a/, /o/, /u/). The letters in our alphabet that can be vowel sounds are *a*, *e*, *i*, *o*, *u*, and *y*.
- Show the children the three parts of an Oreo cookie and have them identify the middle. Talk about how the class will be listening for the "cream" in words.
- Give examples of consonant–vowel–consonant words (e.g., /b/, /a/, /t/ for "bat"). Have the children guess the middle sound in the word. Provide two more examples with the words "cap" and "nut."
- Use a puppet to guess the middle sound in words (e.g., big, map, cut, hit) provided to the class. Have the puppet guess incorrectly at times, and see if the class can judge the responses.

Literature

Read *If You Give a Mouse a Cookie* by Laura Joffe Numeroff.

- Have the children predict what the mouse will want in the book. Use some of the predictions to point out middle sounds in words (e.g., nap, book, name, tape).
- For example, one of the lines in the story is "When the picture is finished, he'll want to sign his name" (/n/, /a/ [long sound], /m/). The middle sound in that word is /a/.

Whole-Class Activity

Preparation

- A "Hot Potato" game, a bean bag, or another such object to pass around is needed. Also, if you do not use the "Hot Potato" game that makes music, you will need a radio or an audiocassette player so that the music can be turned on and off.

Activity

The children will play a game of "Hot Potato."

- The children pass the hot potato or other object around the circle until the music stops. The child who has the hot potato or object when the music stops receives a word from the teacher. The child determines the middle sound in the word.
- Sample words for the whole-class activity include log, miss, bus, fan, win, leaf, bag, hit, run, cat, cup, pat, pet, top, kid, pop, tub, bit, bat, net, cub, mug, pen, and sat.
- For example, "John, what is the sound in the middle of the word 'cub'?" If John responds with /k/, say "/k/ is the first sound in the word 'cub.' What is the middle sound?"

Small-Group Activity

Preparation

- Copy and cut apart paper cookie pieces with letters on them. Consonants can be copied onto light brown paper to represent the outside of the cookies.

Activity

- Place two outside pieces of a paper Oreo-like cookie in the middle of the table for the children to see. One piece will have the first letter (sound) of a word and the other piece will have the last letter (sound) of the word. The teacher has the middle cream part with a vowel on it.
- The teacher says two different vowel sounds while showing two different letters on the cream and asks the child to choose the correct middle sound.
- For example, the child sees two outside pieces, "b" and "g." The teacher reviews the consonant sounds with the children. While showing the two middle letter choices, say "I have an *a* that says the sound /a/ and a *u* that says the sound /u/. Which one do you need to put in the middle to make the word 'bug'?" If the child does not respond correctly, model the sounds again. If the child still does not respond correctly, stress the middle sound in the word. Ask other children to help those children who might struggle. Keep in mind that the children do not need to know all letter and sound matches. The letters are just to accompany the sounds.
- Repeat the steps using new "outside" cookie pieces. Allow enough time for each child to respond at least once. Go through this as many times as needed. The following words may be used in this activity: bag, bug, big, cat, cut, hat, hit, hut, pan, pin, map, bat, bit.

Optional Related Activities

Provide mini-Oreos to children for snack time. Have the children or small group of children determine middle sounds in words to receive the cookies.

- Further expand by seeing if they can identify the beginning, middle, and final sounds in the words.

Materials Needed

Reproducible materials accompanying the lesson:

- Paper cookie pieces for the small-group lesson.

Other materials:

- Paper Oreo-like cookies for the introduction and the small-group activity.
- The "Hot Potato" game or some other object to pass around for the whole-class activity.
- Puppet for the introduction.
- Music to play and turn off during the whole-class activity (if the "Hot Potato" game is not used).

Oreo-like Cookie Pieces for the Small-Group Activity (Lesson 15)

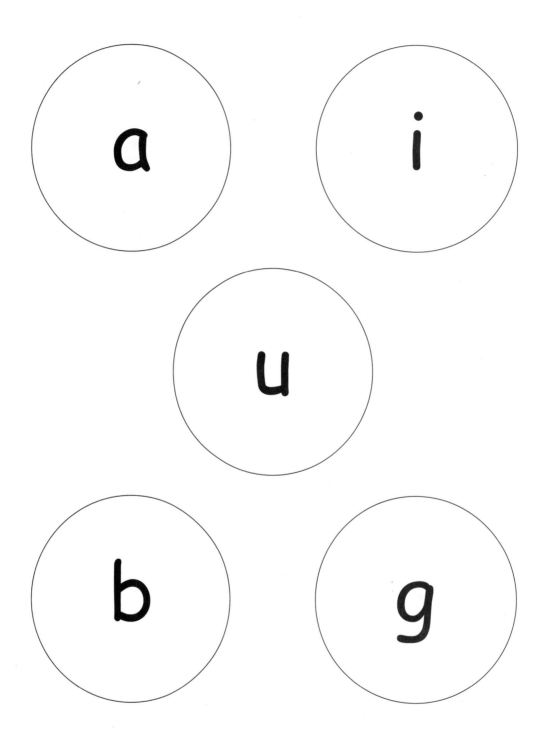

Oreo-like Cookie Pieces for the Small-Group Activity (Lesson 15)

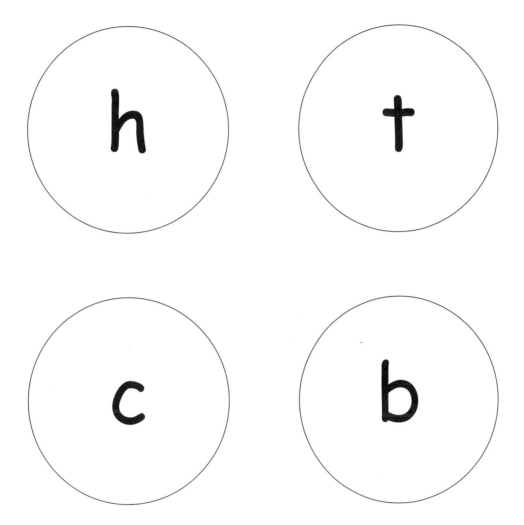

Oreo-like Cookie Pieces for the Small-Group Activity (Lesson 15)

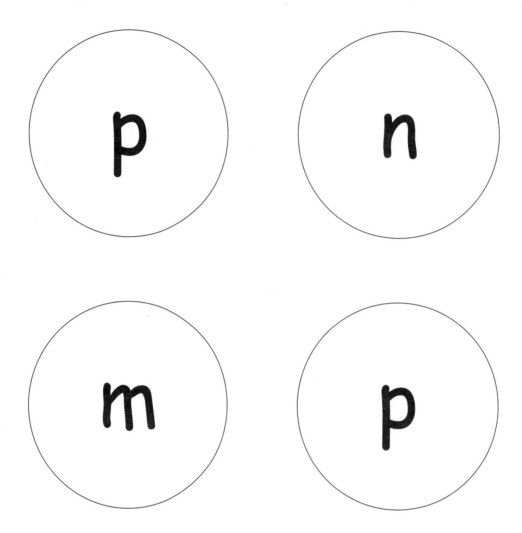

Lesson 16: Phoneme Counting

Introduction

Explain that the class is going to talk about the sounds at the beginning, middle, and end of words and begin to count them to see how many sounds are in certain words.

- Review activities that concentrated on identifying the beginning, middle, and final sounds of words. Make comparisons to the Oreo cookie cream for the middle of words, the caboose of the train for the final sounds, etc. For example, "Class, today we are going to count sounds in words. Some words have two sounds, some have three, four, or more. Let's see if you can guess how many sounds the word 'dig' has." "That's right—'dig' has three sounds. The engine or first sound is /d/, the middle sound is /i/, and the caboose or last sound is /g/."
- Give a few examples of words and see if the children can count on their fingers the number of sounds in those words (e.g., b-u-g = 3; b-y = 2; s-t-o-p = 4). You might use children's names to count number of sounds. If a child responds that his or her name has five sounds when it only has four (e.g., S-t-e-ve = 4 sounds; 5 letters), discuss that concept briefly. "Sometimes words have more sounds than letters and sometimes words have more letters than sounds. That is why we are completing some of these fun word activities to help you learn the similarities and differences between sounds and letters. Today we want to listen carefully to count the number of sounds in words."

Literature

Read *Jump Frog Jump* by Robert Kalan.

- Ask the children to count the number of sounds in the words in the title of the book. (e.g., j-u-m-p = 4; f-r-o-g = 4).
- Stop randomly, say a word from the book, and ask the children which sound is in different parts of the word (e.g., "hop"—What is the first sound in hop?). Emphasize that sound.

Whole-Class Activity

Preparation

- Place four green towels or green paper (make-believe lily pads) in a row.

Activity

- Have one child stand on each lily pad. The rest of the children are in a single-file line by the fourth lily pad.
- Explain that "we are going to jump like frogs to see how many sounds are in some of the words we are going to talk about."

- You will be saying a word and then saying the individual sounds of the word. The class will help you determine the sounds in the word. For example, if the word is "sad," you will say the word, point to the first child on the first lily pad and tell him or her to get ready to produce /s/. Place your hand on the shoulder of the first child and have him or her say the sound. Once the sound is said, the child jumps like a frog off the lily pad. Then, you point to the second child and put your mouth in the position for the vowel sound. Have the second child say the sound. Again, after the sound is produced, the child jumps off the lily pad. Continue with the last sound and then say the word "sad."
- Count the number of sounds in each word after the children have jumped: "There are three sounds in the word 'sad,' /s/, /a/, /d/."
- Ask the children in line to raise their hands to tell the class how many sounds are in each word (e.g., s-a-d = 3 sounds). You should exaggerate each sound and count with fingers to show the class the number of sounds.
- Have each child move up one lily pad. The child standing on the first lily pad will go to the end of the line. The child standing on the fourth lily pad will move to the first lily pad.
- Words for Whole-Class Activity:

Two-Phoneme Words	Three-Phoneme Words	Four-Phoneme Words
pea	bat	plate
ice	rain	great
pay	nail	stone
say	lake	plane
pie	rice	slime
ache	pill	flake
egg	cup	spoon
ate	nut	spice

Small-Group Activity

Preparation

- Copy a frog picture for each child. A Popsicle stick or tongue blade for each child and glue are also needed for the activity.

Activity

Have each child glue a frog drawing onto a tongue blade or Popsicle stick. Use the above words from the whole-class lesson to complete the following tasks:

- First round: Say a word and have all the children identify the first sound. (The children can have their frog say the sounds.)
- Second round: Say a word and have all the children identify the final sound.
- Third round: Explain that you will sound out each word (exaggerate each sound) and have a child tell you how many sounds the child heard. If he or she has difficulty, then count the sounds on your fingers. The child should make the frog hop that many times. For example, if

the word was "map," the frog would hop at /m/, /a/, and /p/ and say "three." Give each child a chance to figure it out alone before allowing the other children to help.

- After providing the children with the word "ice," say "Make the frog hop for each sound in the word 'ice.' How many times should the frog jump?"
- If a child has difficulty, say the word together slowly. Consider placing your hand on the child's wrist and making the frog hop as you say the sounds.

Optional Related Activities

Write the numbers 2, 3, and 4 on the chalkboard. Draw lines to separate the numbers.

- Give the children a word and have them identify how many sounds are in the word. Have a child come to the front of the room to make a mark in the appropriate column.
- Have the children crouch down like frogs. Name a word, then say each sound in that word, jumping after the sound is produced. The teacher can jump too. Ask the class, "How many times did we jump?" "Yes, we jumped three times because 'grow' has three sounds."

Materials Needed

Reproducible materials accompanying the lesson:

- Frog drawings to glue on Popsicle sticks or tongue blades for the small-group activity.

Other materials:

- Book: *Jump Frog Jump* by Robert Kalan. New York: Greenwillow Books, 1981. ISBN: 0-688-13954-X.
- Green towels (make-believe lily pads) for the whole-class activity.
- Tongue blades or Popsicle sticks for the small-group activity.
- Glue for the small-group activity.

Picture of a Frog for the Small-Group Activity (Lesson 16)

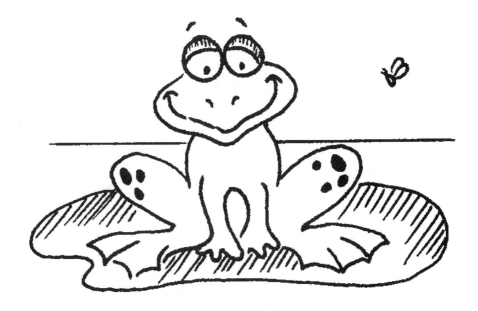

Lesson 17: Blending Two- and Three-Phoneme Word

Introduction

Discuss the concept of blending, which is listening to each sound and putting the sounds together to make words: "Boys and girls, today we are going to listen very carefully for each sound in a word and put them together to see what the word is. Let's try one together. Listen carefully: /g/, /u/, /m/. Does anyone know what word those sounds make?"

- Provide the sounds /m/, /a/, /t/, pausing between each sound. Ask the class to guess what word it is. See if anyone can guess what the sounds /s/, /i/, /t/ make. Try another one: /u/, /p/. Provide some more examples for the children (/i/, /ce/; /b/, /a/, /g/).
- Once the children guess the word, say the sounds again separately, then reinforce the word they chose: "Yes, the sounds /i/, /ce/ make the word 'ice.' That word has two sounds in it."

Literature

Read *One Fish, Two Fish, Red Fish, Blue Fish* by Dr. Seuss.

- Introduce the title of the book, but pause before the word "blue" and say the individual sounds (/b/, /l/, /ue/). Ask the children what word that was.
- After reading the book, go back through it and find different words. Say the sounds of a word and have the children guess what word you are sounding out.
- Sample words to use include the following: fish (/f/, /i/, /sh/); red (/r/, /e/, /d/); sad (/s/, /a/, /d/); two (/t/, /wo/); feet (/f/, /ee/, /t/); bump (/b/, /u/, /m/, /p/); head (/h/, /ea/, /d/); house (/h/, /ou/, /se/).
- Consider using contextual cues such as "One fish, t—wo"; the children may guess "two."

Whole-Class Activity

Preparation

Copy and cut apart the fish word cards provided. Place a paper clip on each card. You will also need a fishing pole with a magnet attached to it and a bag or container to hold the fish when caught.

Activity

This activity involves the children using the magnetic fishing pole to catch fish (word cards) from a make-believe pond. The fish have two- or three-phoneme words written on them.

- The children form a circle to get ready to fish from the pond.
- Have one child at a time use the fishing pole to catch a fish.
- The teacher takes the fish off the magnet and says the phonemes of the word on the fish, and

the child names the word. For example, if the word on a fish is "bug," the teacher will say /b/, /u/, /g/.

- If the child does not understand, repeat the sounds. Also, consider combining the rime portion of the word /b/, /ug/ to help the child. If the child still has difficulty, use a clue such as "it is an insect, like a fly." If the child needs additional help, ask another child.
- Have each child take a turn, and then put their fish in a bag, net, or other container after catching it. The child will go back to the circle and possibly take another turn if time allows.

Small-Group Activity

Preparation

Copy and cut apart the small-group picture cards.

Activity

Play a variation of a "Go Fish" game.

- Each child will get four picture cards. The following pictures are included for the "Go Fish" game: pig, wig, lip, rip, sheep, sleep, bug, hug, mop, top, house, mouse, whale, sail, toe, bow, pie, knee, tea, ice, key, up, bye, and egg.
- You say the sounds of each word with a pause between each sound of the word: for example, sheep—"sh-ee-p."
- The children will try to guess the word and then determine if one of their pictures matches the word that the teacher said (not every child will have a picture that matches, so the children will have to determine if any of their pictures match the word).
- When the child makes a match, he or she will give the picture card to the teacher.
- Repeat until all matches are made. Reshuffle and play the game again if time allows.
- If the children are having difficulty, say the onsets and rimes of the words to assist them.

Optional Related Activities

When singing familiar songs in the classroom, stop at the end of a line to blend phonemes together and see if the children can guess the word. This activity should give the children a sense of success since they may be familiar with the verses in the song. For example, when singing "Five Little Ducks," sing "Five little ducks went out one /d/, /ay/."

Materials Needed

Reproducible materials accompanying the lesson:

- Fish shapes with words on them for the whole-class activity.
- Picture cards for the small-group activity.

Other materials:

- Book: *One Fish, Two Fish, Red Fish, Blue Fish* by Dr. Seuss. New York: Random House, 1988. ISBN: 0-394-90013-8.
- A small make-believe pond (a large piece of blue paper or small swimming pool).
- A fishing pole with a magnet at the end for the whole-class activity.
- A bag, net, or container to hold the fish for the whole-class activity.

Words for Whole-Class Activity (Lesson 17)

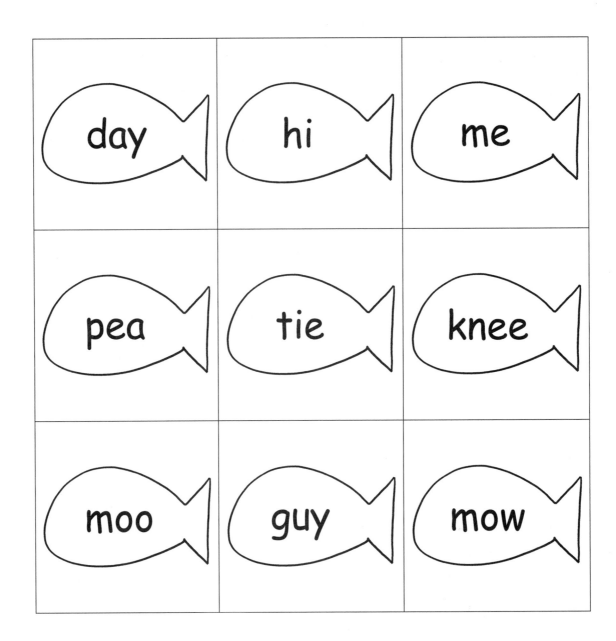

Words for Whole-Class Activity (Lesson 17)

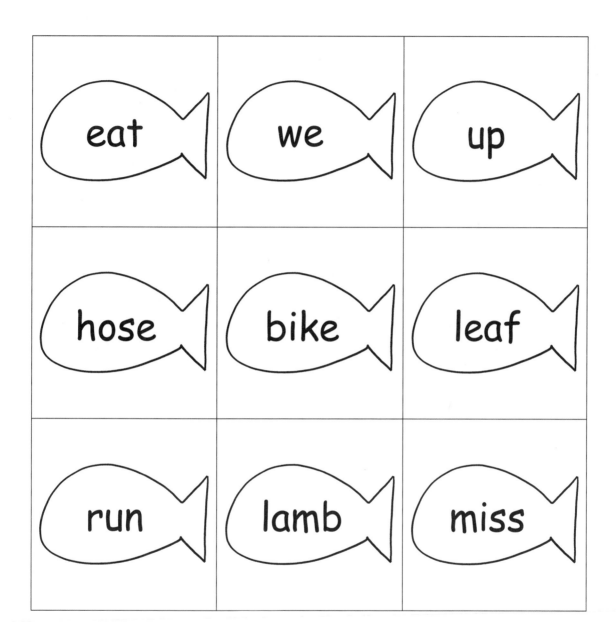

Words for Whole-Class Activity (Lesson 17)

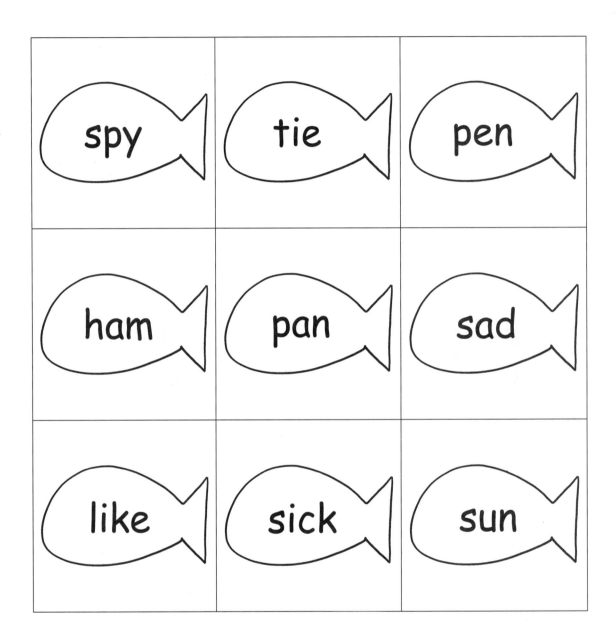

Small-Group Picture Cards (Lesson 17)

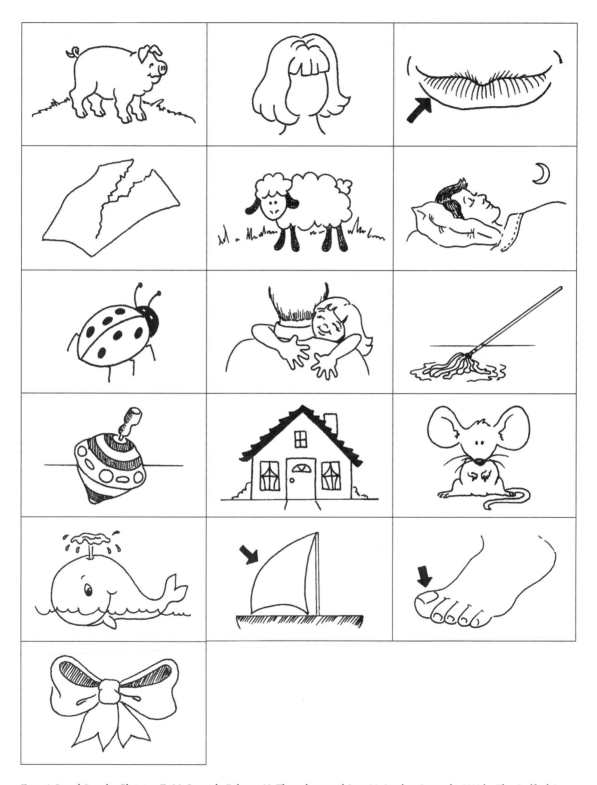

Small-Group Picture Cards (Lesson 17)

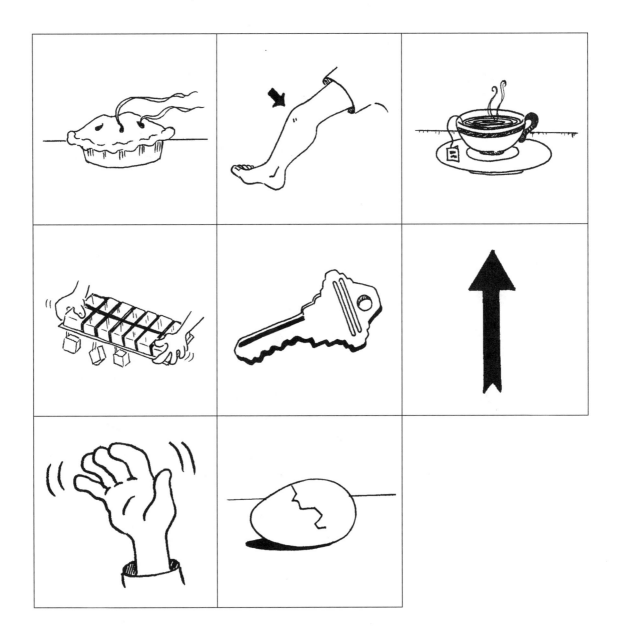

Lesson 18: Phoneme Blending

Introduction

Review the concept of blending. "Listen very carefully to the sounds I say and tell me what this word is: /zzz/, pause /i/, pause /p/. Who can guess what that word was?"

- Write some simple words on the board to show the children how when you put the letters *z*, *i*, *p* together, the sounds of these letters make the word "zip."
- Turn off the lights in the classroom and make it as dark as possible. Tell the children we will shortly be reading a book about a turtle. Ask them to crouch down on their knees and place their heads toward the floor, pretending they are turtles. Explain that you will be saying sounds of a word and if they think they know the answer, to come out of their shells. The teacher will shine a flashlight on the child as a signal to say the answer.
- Walk around the class behind the children, next to them, and in front of them to build suspense. If they get uncomfortable with their heads in their laps, have them cover their eyes with their hands. Sample words include pack (/p/, /a/, /ck/), bell, wet, red, lock, hug, win.

Literature

Read *Franklin in the Dark* by Paulette Bourgeois and Brenda Clark.

- Pause before the final word in some sentences and sound out the word. Let the children guess what the word was. For example, read one of the sentences on page 6 of the book: "Every night, Franklin's mother would take a flashlight and shine it into his /sh/ (*pause*), /e/ (*pause*), /l/." Children then are given time to guess "shell."

Whole-Class Activity

Preparation

A bedsheet is needed.

Activity

The children will be pretending they are turtles by peeking their heads out from behind a sheet to say a sound provided by the teacher. The rest of the class will guess the word.

- Have two children help hold the sheet for their classmates.
- Explain to the class that children called to come behind the sheet will pretend they are turtles. They will peek their heads over the sheet (out of their shells) to say a sound aloud. Be sure to remind the children to say the sound after the class can see their heads: "The class might need some clues from your mouths to guess the sounds."
- Call three children to come behind the sheet. Whisper a sound into each of their ears (e.g.,

/sh/, /o/, /p/). Have them poke their heads over the sheet and say the sound clearly to see if the class can guess the word.

- Continue with other children. It may be necessary to repeat the sounds for the class. Sample words include get, men, jet, pen, rub, hit, tug, rice, gate, hop, lake, coat, and rose.

Small-Group Activity

Preparation

Cut apart the turtle pictures included with this lesson and place them in a small box.

Activity

- Begin the activity by placing three or four pictures from the box in front of the child. Say the sounds of the word matching one of the pictures, and see if the child picks the right picture. When the child guesses the word, he or she gets to keep the turtle with the picture on it. Let each child have a turn completing the activity with picture choices.
- Continue the activity by placing all the turtles back in the box. Choose a turtle out of the box and say the sounds of the word matching the picture. If the child guesses the word, he or she gets to keep the picture. Proceed around the circle until all children have taken four or five turns. If time allows, place the pictures back in the box and play again.

Optional Related Activities

Pause before providing a word to the class for directions to an activity. For example, "Children, we need pipe cleaners and (*pause*) /b/, /ea/, /d/, /z/ (beads) for this activity. Can anyone guess what it is we need to go with the pipe cleaners?" Another example: "Who needs a little bit of /w/, /a/, /t/, /er/? Let's line up to get a drink."

Materials Needed

Reproducible materials accompanying the lesson:

- Turtle pictures cut apart for the small-group activity.

Other materials:

- Book: *Franklin in the Dark* by Paulette Bourgeois and Brenda Clark. New York: Scholastic, 1986. ISBN: 0-590-44506-5.
- A flashlight for the introduction.
- A sheet for the whole-class activity.
- A small box for the small-group activity.

Turtle Pictures for the Small-Group Activity (Lesson 18)

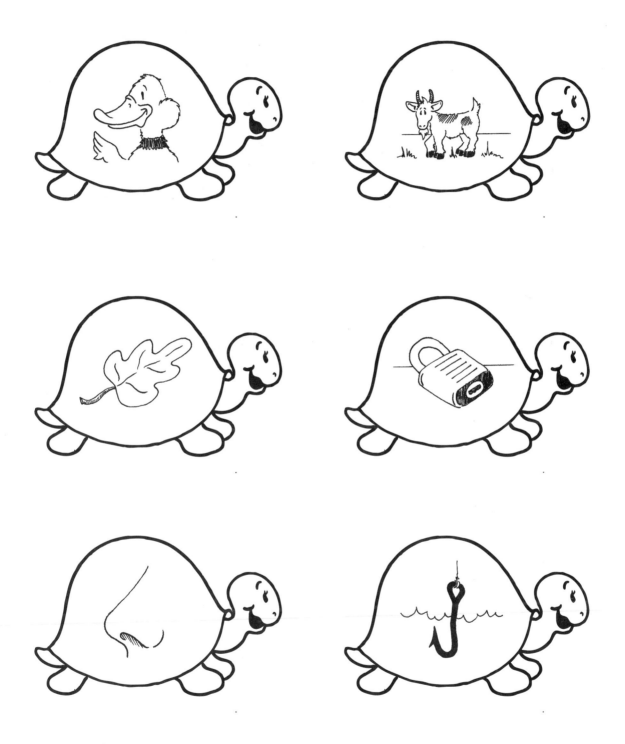

Turtle Pictures for the Small-Group Activity (Lesson 18)

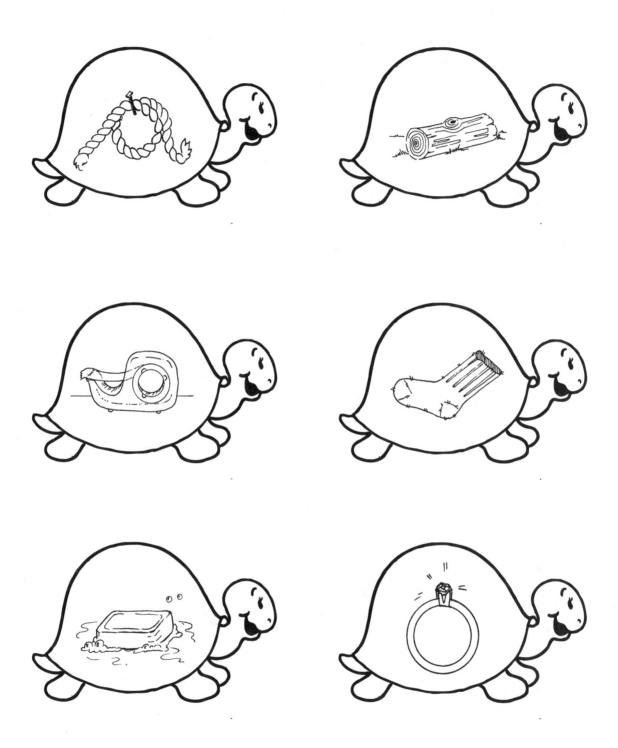

Turtle Pictures for the Small-Group Activity (Lesson 18)

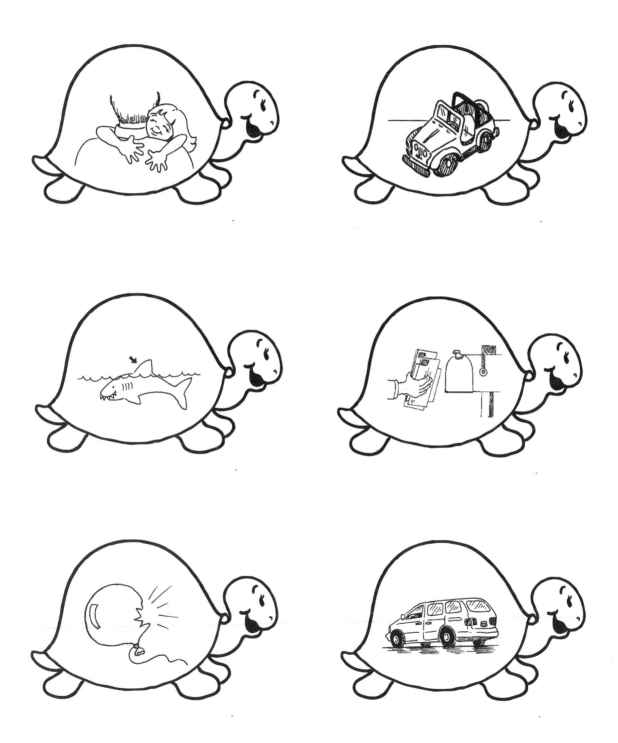

Pictures for the Small-Group Activity (Lesson 18)

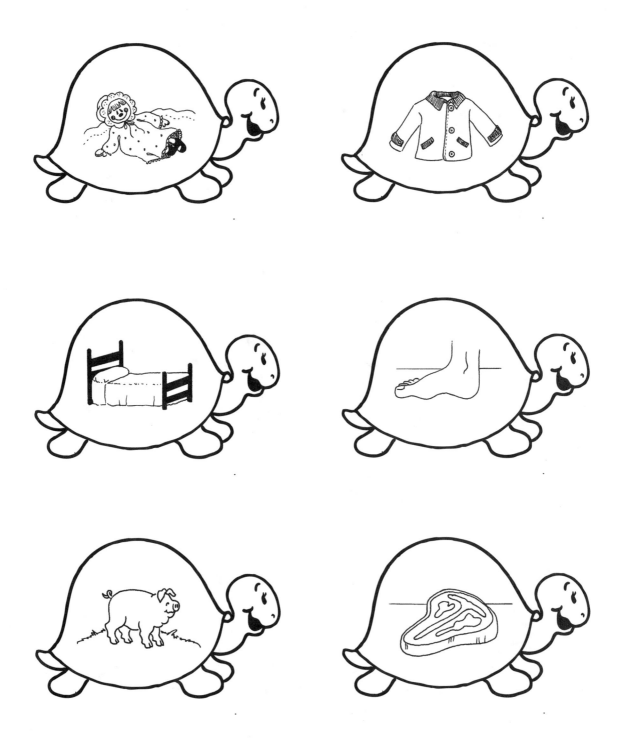

Lesson 19: Phoneme Segmentation

Introduction

Preparation

Copy the introduction words included with this lesson, and cut them apart from each other.

Activity

Explain the concept of phoneme segmentation to the class: "Last week we listened carefully to sounds and put them together to make a word. This week, we are going to figure out the sounds that are in words. For example, I'm thinking of a word that is the name of something in the sky—it is yellow and bright; does anyone know what it might be? . . . Yes, it is the sun. Let's try to figure out the sounds in the word 'sun.' What is the first sound? . . . Yes, it's /s/. What is the second sound? . . . Yes it's /u/. What is the third sound? Yes, it's /n/. When we break apart the word sun, we have /s/, /u/, /n/."

- Use the visual words incorporated with this lesson. Show the children the printed word, and tell them what the word is. For example: "Children, this word is 'map.' Help me break apart this word by saying the sounds in the word slowly. As we say each sound, I will cut the sound off with scissors. The first sound in 'map' is /m/. Cut it off. The next sound is /a/. Cut it off. The last sound is /p/. Cut it off. We took the word 'map' and broke it apart into its sounds: /m/, /a/, /p/ are the sounds in the word 'map.' "
- Complete a couple more examples in front of the class. Consider having a child come to the front of the class to help you figure out the sounds in the word.
- Another idea is to write words on the board and have children come forward to erase the letters as they say the sounds. Use consonant–vowel–consonant words that are phonetically appropriate (e.g., sad, dig, man, top). If the class seems to be catching on fairly well, provide a few examples of words that are more difficult (e.g., meat, chop, mine). Erase or cut apart two letters that make one sound and explain to the children that sometimes more than one letter is needed to make one sound.

Literature

Read *Big Sarah's Little Boots* by Paulette Bourgeois and Brenda Clark.

- Choose a few words in the book to segment for the class. For example, the last word on page 4 of the above book is "feet." Read the last sentence: "But Sarah's boots did not fit Sarah's feet" (/f/, /ee/, /t/).
- Another example is in the sentence on page 9: "They tied one end of the boots to Matthew's horse and the other end to Sarah's bike" (/b/, /i/, /ke/).

Whole-Class Activity

Preparation

Put five chairs in front of the class. Place dolls or stuffed animals on the chairs.

Activity

Demonstrate for the class how the dolls or stuffed animals are going to tell us the sounds in words and break words apart. Tell the children to listen carefully because some words have two sounds, some have three, some have four, and some have none.

- Use the following word lists for this activity:

Two-sound words	Three-sound words	Four-sound words	Five- or six-sound words
shoe	boat	baby	stamp
tie	dog	cookie	video
tea	hat	glove	kickoff
ape	phone	penny	slimy
egg	book	zipper	police
boy	sock	snake	salad
egg	tape	frog	bucket
pie	ball	block	peanut
ice	mice	slice	rainbow
ill	will	spill	raccoon
us	bus	twin	cracker

- Stand the dolls up on the chairs. Say a word to the dolls, and pretend they are thinking about the sounds in the word. Go behind each doll and have the doll sit down as you say each sound. For example, demonstrate a two-sound word by saying the word "tea" to the dolls. Go behind the first doll and pretend that she is thinking about the first sound, then say /t/ and have her sit down; go to the next doll, and say /ea/ and have her sit down. Discuss how that was a short word and only had two sounds. If a child responds that "tea" has three letters, say "That's right! Tea does have three letters—the *ea* makes one sound /ea/. Tea has three letters and two sounds. Good thinking." Do several more words with the dolls.
- Take the dolls off the chairs, and ask the children to come forward to demonstrate the sounds in words. Have the children stand while you give them a word to think about. Remind them that they might not all have a sound with each word. Ask five children to come forward and say the word "pillow" (/p/, /i/, /ll/, /ow/). See if the first child can think of the first sound in the word; proceed through the word. Stand behind each of the children, and place your hand on his or her shoulder as each says a sound and then sits. When they are finished, have the fifth child move to the first chair and four more children come forward.

Small-Group Activity

Preparation

Use small Unifix cubes that interlock and the word lists included above for this activity.

Activity

- Provide each child with a stack of six Unifix cubes. Give the children a word and have them take a cube off for each sound in the word. When finished, ask them to count the number of cubes they took off. Compare and discuss the responses. For example, if you gave the children the word, "bet," they should each have taken off three cubes. Review the sounds by pointing to a cube and saying the individual sounds in the word.
- After a few group trials, go around the table and ask each child to complete this activity while the others watch and listen.

Optional Related Activities

Have the children jump to the sounds in words provided to them. For example, have all the children stand. Say a word to the class and have them jump one time for each sound in the word. Another gross motor activity may also be used (e.g., bouncing a ball, clapping, snapping fingers).

Materials Needed

Reproducible materials accompanying the lesson:

- The words printed on the accompanying form, which is to be cut apart for the introduction.

Other materials:

- Book: *Big Sarah's Little Boots* by Paulette Bourgeois and Brenda Clark. Scholastic, 1987. ISBN: 0-590-42623-0.
- Scissors for the introduction.
- Dolls or stuffed animals (5) for the whole-class activity.
- Five small chairs for the whole-class activity.
- Unifix cubes for the small-group activity.

Introduction Words (Lesson 19)

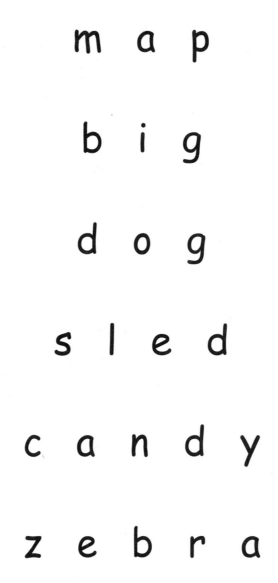

m a p

b i g

d o g

s l e d

c a n d y

z e b r a

Lesson 20: Review of Initial, Medial, and Final Sounds and of Phoneme Counting, Blending, and Segmenting

Introduction

Explain that many things are going to be reviewed that the children have been learning about sounds and words.

- Discuss the skills we have targeted from the beginning of Lesson 11: "Children, we learned to listen for the first sound in words, the last sound in words, and that some words have middle sounds. We listened very carefully to those sounds to form words. Sometimes those words had two sounds, three sounds, four sounds or more. You know so much about sounds and words that I want to put everything together today to see how much you have learned."
- Give some examples of the above skills. Tell them they need to listen very carefully to the questions because they might be tricky:

  1. "What is the first sound in 'bug'?"
  2. "What is another word that starts with the same first sound as 'cat'?"
  3. "What is the last sound in 'pan'?"
  4. "What word do these sounds make: /c/, /a/, /ke/?"
  5. "Listen carefully to this word: 'baby.' Who can tell me the sounds in the word 'baby'?"
  6. "Does the word 'dog' have a middle sound? Who can tell me what the sound is?"

Literature

Read *It Begins with an A* by Stephanie Calmenson.

- Let the children guess the objects on each page. Emphasize and exaggerate the production of the first sound after the children guess. For example, when they guess 'nose,' say, "That's right. You smell with your nnnnnnose."
- Continue to ask other questions from the book that review all the skills targeted the last several weeks. For example, after the children guess 'foot,' ask how many sounds the word 'foot' has. Ask the children what the middle sound in the word 'moon' is. Ask the children what the last sound in 'ball' is. Ask the children what this word is: /s/, /a/, /d/ = sad.

Whole-Class Activity

Preparation

Cut apart the questions included at the end of this lesson and put a question strip in plastic eggs. Hide the eggs around the room or outside for each child in the class to find two.

Activity

- Explain to the class that "we are going to have our own egg hunt." Feel free to conduct this hunt outside or in the classroom (or another available room in the building with more space). The children are instructed to find one egg and then sit back down, line up to go inside, etc. without opening the egg. Have the children sit in an egg shape on the floor.
- The teacher will open an egg in front of the class. The teacher will model what she wants the children to do. Open an egg and read this question to the class: "What is the first sound in the word 'farm'?" and the class will respond.
- Go around the class and one at a time, have each child open the egg and answer the question you read from the strip of paper.
- When the child is finished, have him or her put the egg in a basket placed in the middle of the circle.
- Feel free to use the chart attached to this lesson to collect data on the questions asked for an informal assessment. You will not be able to collect all data on each child but can get a sample from children.

Small-Group Activity

Complete a similar activity to the large-group activity.

- Place the eggs with a sentence strip in them in a basket and place the basket in the middle of the table. Go around the circle and have each child choose an egg.
- Use the chart attached to this unit to keep track of the children's responses. Try to ask the children at least two questions from each category on the chart.
- An alteration might be to place a few pieces of candy in some of the eggs. Each child might be limited to two eggs with candy in them. This might maintain their interest and motivation to listen.

Optional Related Activities

Sing the song "The Big White Bunny Found a Basket" to the tune of "Old McDonald Had a Farm":

- The Big White Bunny found a basket
    Egg-I-egg-I-O
  And in that basket was a /d/ (*change sounds each verse*)
    Egg-I-egg-I-O
  With a duck duck here and a duck duck there
  Here a duck, there a duck, everywhere a duck, duck
  The Big White Bunny found a basket
    Egg-I-egg-I-O

  (*Replace "duck" with other words depending on the sound inserted.*)

Materials Needed

Reproducible materials accompanying the lesson:

- Question strips for eggs for the whole-class and small-group activities.
- Data chart for the whole-class (optional) and small-group activities.

Other materials:

- Book: *It Begins with an A* by Stephanie Calmenson. New York: Scholastic, 1994. ISBN: 0-590-48173-8.
- Plastic eggs for the whole-class and small-group activities.

Questions for Whole-Class and Small-Group Activities (Lesson 20)

INITIAL SOUND

- What is the first sound in "ball"?
- What is another word that starts with the same first sound as in "ball"?
- What is the first sound in "phone"?
- What is another word that starts with the same first sound as in "phone"?
- What is the first sound in "run"?
- What is another word that starts with the same first sound as in "run"?
- What is the first sound in "milk"?
- What is another word that starts with the same first sound as in "milk"?
- What is the first sound in "toe"?
- What is another word that starts with the same first sound as in "toe"?

MEDIAL SOUND

- What is the middle sound in "boat"?
- What is the middle sound in "fine"?
- What is the middle sound in "game"?
- What is the middle sound in "seat"?
- What is the middle sound in "room"?
- What is the middle sound in "dot"?
- What is the middle sound in "nose"?
- What is the middle sound in "cut"?
- What is the middle sound in "web"?
- What is the middle sound in "take"?

FINAL SOUND

- What is the last sound in "bike"?
- What is another word that ends with the same last sound as in "bike"?
- What is the last sound in "fun"?
- What is another word that ends with the same last sound as in "fun"?
- What is the last sound in "pail"?
- What is another word that ends with the same last sound as in "pail"?
- What is the last sound in "bug"?
- What is another word that ends with the same last sound as in "bug"?
- What is the last sound in "nap"?
- What is another word that ends with the same last sound as in "nap"?

PHONEME COUNTING

- How many sounds are in the word "see"?
- How many sounds are in the word "bye"?
- How many sounds are in the word "day"?
- How many sounds are in the word "coat"?
- How many sounds are in the word "game"?
- How many sounds are in the word "rug"?
- How many sounds are in the word "sad"?
- How many sounds are in the word "happy"?
- How many sounds are in the word "bunny"?
- How many sounds are in the word "cookie"?

PHONEME SEGMENTATION

- Tell me the sounds in the word "fish."
- Tell me the sounds in the word "night."
- Tell me the sounds in the word "date."
- Tell me the sounds in the word "pop."
- Tell me the sounds in the word "gum."
- Tell me the sounds in the word "rock."
- Tell me the sounds in the word "meat."
- Tell me the sounds in the word "joke."
- Tell me the sounds in the word "lamb."
- Tell me the sounds in the word "kite."

PHONEME BLENDING

- What word do these sounds make: /m/, /o/, /m/?
- What word do these sounds make: /g/, /oa/, /t/?
- What word do these sounds make: /s/, /a/, /ck/?
- What word do these sounds make: /b/, /oo/, /k/?
- What word do these sounds make: /c/, /a/, /t/?
- What word do these sounds make: /n/, /ai/, /l/?
- What word do these sounds make: /t/, /a/, /p/?
- What word do these sounds make: /l/, /igh/, /t/?
- What word do these sounds make: /d/, /o/, /g/?
- What word do these sounds make: /f/, /ee/, /t/?

Data Chart (Lesson 20)

Date _____

Child's name	Initial sound	Medial sound	Final sound	Phoneme counting	Phoneme blending	Phoneme segmenting

Chapter 4

Individualized Instruction in Phonemic Awareness

Providing class instruction on phonemic awareness skills through fun and engaging class activities is a major step toward helping all children get off to a good start in reading. However, while the majority of children will demonstrate substantial progress on these skills, it is likely that some children will be having difficulty catching on to the awareness of phonemes. From our experience, which is consistent with the findings of Torgesen (2000), around 5% children will still have difficulty with phoneme awareness even with whole-class and small-group instruction. These children are at risk for developing reading difficulties because it is the phoneme level of phonemic awareness skills that is most directly related to understanding how our alphabet works to represent sounds in print (Adams, Treiman, & Pressley, 1998).

As noted in Chapter 1, children vary in their general language development and their ability to process phonological information—that is, to process spoken language. Phonological processing skills are reflected in the ease with which children develop skills of phonemic awareness and letter knowledge. Limited general language development and impaired phonological processing skills can interfere with learning to read because letter knowledge, phonemic awareness, and the ease with which these skills are learned are all highly predictive of success in learning to read (Torgesen et al., 1999; Byrne, Fielding-Barnsley, & Ashley, 2000).

How many children in a class are not catching on to phoneme awareness after explicit teaching of these skills varies with the class. It may be that only one or two children are having difficulty with phonemes, or it may be that a larger number of children are having difficulty. This number is highly influenced by young children's language experiences and the individual differences among the children. Providing more intensive and explicit teaching of the skills directly related to the alphabetic principle can improve the at-risk child's likelihood of success with learning to read (National Reading Panel, 2000; Chard & Dickson, 1999; Torgesen et al., 1999).

Chard and Dickson (1999) refer to this more intensive level as second-tier instruction and provide research-based guidelines for this instruction. The lessons that follow in Chapter 5 are consistent with their recommendations: (1) The lessons focus on the phoneme level. (2) They provide appropriate practice in identifying phonemes within words. (3) They include matching specific phonemes to specific letters. For some children this individualized instruction will be sufficient preparation for beginning reading instruction. However, as Torgesen (2000) points out, some children may need continued intensive instructional support throughout the elementary years.

THE INDIVIDUALIZED LESSONS

The individualized (or second-tier) lessons in Chapter 5 are appropriate for the second semester of kindergarten or first semester of first-grade with children who have received class instruction in phonemic awareness skills but are not developing skills in identifying individual sounds within words. The sequence of lessons focuses on skills directly predictive of learning to decode. Remember that these skills are not the only important skills for learning to read, and the children should continue with class activities that include phonemic awareness, letter knowledge skills, shared book reading, and language enrichment.

Because the focus of these lessons is on helping the at-risk child to understand and begin to use the alphabetic principle, beginning and ending phonemes are taught as well as their matching letters. The teacher models the instructional task before the child attempts it and, if necessary, guides the child toward a correct response. This approach of continually providing corrective feedback also allows the greatest possibility of the child's success with each lesson. Each lesson should provide a positive and enjoyable experience for each child.

The 16 lessons are presented in sessions of around 15 minutes each. They can be presented in approximately 8 weeks with two sessions each week or adapted to your class schedule. The directions were developed for individualized instruction, the instructional approach used by Torgesen et al. (1999) with at-risk children. However, you can readily use the lessons with two or three children. The length of sessions and number of sessions are flexible, depending on the needs of the individual children.

The lessons begin with identifying phonemes at the beginning of spoken words and then introduce the letter which corresponds to that phoneme. The letters are introduced early because having a concrete representation of the phoneme can provide a helpful additional support (Chard & Dickson, 1999; Adams et al., 1998). A small set of six phonemes (and their corresponding letters) at the beginning and end of words is used throughout the lessons. The six phonemes (/m/, /s/, /f/, /n/, /p/, /t/) used in the lessons begin with phonemes which can be prolonged or drawn out (/m/, /s/, /f/, /n/) and are thus easy to identify. The set of six phonemes allows an adequate number of words for practice in the lessons. Vowel phonemes (and letters) are not included because medial sounds are much more difficult to hear than beginning and ending sounds and may not be essential to begin reading instruction (Torgesen & Mathes, 2000). When the lessons involve segmenting and blending sounds, only three phoneme words are used in order to provide maximum support for acquiring these skills.

Sequence of lessons:

Pretest
1. Beginning Sounds /m/ and /s/
2. Beginning Sounds /f/ and /n/
3. Beginning Sounds /p/ and /t/
4. Review of Beginning Sounds
5. Letters *m* and *s* for Beginning Sounds
6. Letters *f* and *n* for Beginning Sounds
7. Letters *p* and *t* for Beginning Sounds
8. Letters *m*, *s*, and *f* for Beginning Sounds
9. Letters *n*, *p*, and *t* for Beginning Sounds
10. Review of Letters for Beginning Sounds

11. Letters /n/, /p/, /t/ for Ending Sounds
12. Ending Sounds /n/, /p/, /t/
13. Ending Sounds /n/, /p/, /t/
14. Beginning Letters *m, s, f* and Ending Letters *n, p, t*
15. Beginning Letters *n, p, t* and Ending Letters *n, p, t*
16. Letters for Beginning and Ending Sounds
Posttest and Take-Home Tiny Books

ASSESSMENT FOR THE INDIVIDUALIZED LESSONS

Assessment of awareness of phonemes is used in two ways with these lessons (the procedure is explained in the *Getting Started* section later in this chapter):

First, assessment is used to identify children showing minimal progress on phoneme awareness. The *Test of Phonological Awareness* (TOPA), Kindergarten Version, (Torgesen & Bryant, 1994) is recommended to identify those children who are not progressing midway in the kindergarten year. This standardized test can be given to individual children or small groups of children in about 15 minutes. It assesses recognition of beginning sounds and provides both percentile ranks and standard scores.

Second, the informal assessment included in this chapter should be given before Lesson 1 and after Lesson 16 as a means of assessing the progress of each child receiving the individualized instruction. This measure assesses the skills taught in the lessons. Six items assess first sounds in words, six items assess last sounds in words, and six items assess representing first and last sounds in words with letters. Twenty-four points are possible. The test is given individually and takes about 10 minutes. The directions for giving the test and scoring it are included.

EFFECTIVENESS OF THE LESSONS

The lessons in Chapter 5 directly teach the skills recommended for the second tier of instruction by Chard and Dickson (1999). The lessons were written to provide maximal support for the child's developing awareness of specific phonemes and their match to letters at the beginning and end of words. The lessons were refined by using them for several years with kindergarten children who were identified by their teachers as at risk for reading problems in the first grade. The directions, skills, and activities were revised as needed to ensure the likelihood that each child could successfully progress through the sequence of skills presented in the lessons.

For 8 weeks during March and April of 2001, the lessons of Chapter 5 were given individually to four at-risk kindergarten children (Ochs, 2001). The children's progress was assessed weekly using alternative forms of the measure that accompanies the lessons. Prior to beginning the lessons, all four children scored below the 25th percentile on the TOPA (Torgesen & Bryant, 1994) and less than 8 on the pretest assessment for these lessons. As can be seen in Figure 4.1, each child showed improved scores across the weeks of instruction. Three of the four children received the highest possible score (24) on the assessment during the later lessons and, at the conclusion of the lessons, showed average scores on the TOPA between the 55th and 71st percentile. The one child not showing maximum progress, and who still had difficulty with identifying phonemes at the beginning and end of words, scored well below average on the TOPA at the conclusion of the lessons. She was found to be eligible for special education services shortly after the lessons were concluded and will continue to need instructional support in learning to read.

GETTING STARTED

1. The first step is to identify children in need of more intensive, individualized instruction. After class lessons on initial phonemes have been presented (e.g., Lessons 11 and 12 in Chapter 3), those children not demonstrating the skill should be considered for the instruction in these individualized lessons. As a check on your perceptions of which children are not progressing, administer the TOPA, Kindergarten Version (Torgesen & Bryant, 1994), to these children or the entire class. Any child scoring below the 25th percentile should be considered for individualized instruction. (This assessment can also give you information regarding the status of your class as a whole. If many children score below the 25th percentile, then the class would likely benefit from increased whole-class instruction, especially at the phoneme level.)

2. After you have identified the children in step 1, individually administer and score the Assessment for Individualized Lessons found in this chapter, which was developed to accompany the lessons (used for both the pre- and postassessment). If TOPA scores are not available, children who score below 8 on the first two tasks (repeating beginning or ending sounds) are likely to benefit from the lessons.

3. Arrange for a quiet work space for the lessons and schedule a time that does not interfere with other class early reading activities. The lessons can be given by the child's teacher, reading teacher, or speech–language pathologist.

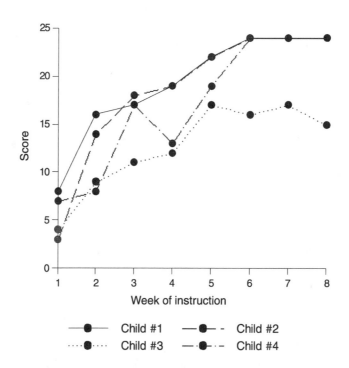

FIGURE 4.1. Individual assessment scores across 8 weeks of lessons.

4. If, on the pretest, beginning sounds can be identified, proceed through the sequence of lessons but omit Activity Pages for Lessons 1–3. In general, present each lesson in sequence. However, if the child clearly has mastered the skills for a lesson, the Activity Page can be omitted.

5. Duplicate and cut materials; if you duplicate the teacher's materials on card stock and keep them in labeled plastic bags or envelopes, they are more durable and can be used many times. The children's materials need to be duplicated for each child. Also assemble a supply of stickers and a glue stick or tape for each child to use with the Activity Pages.

6. Read through the directions for each lesson carefully before beginning the lesson. When reading the directions, be attentive to the difference between the sound of the phoneme (e.g., /m/) and the letter (*m*).

7. Begin each lesson with a friendly comment to the child, and always respond positively to any question or comment from the child. A warm and positive teacher can help to ensure that each child finds the lesson an enjoyable learning experience.

8. Conclude each lesson with a comment about how the child is learning the skills that will help with learning to read; allow the child to select a sticker. Keep track of each child's progress through the lessons on the Progress Chart included at the end of this chapter.

9. At the conclusion of the lessons readminister to each child the informal assessment in this chapter. If the child scores below 24 on this posttest, additional instructional support is likely to be needed in the future.

REFERENCES

Adams, M., Treiman, R., & Pressley M. (1998). Reading, writing and literacy. In I. Siegel & K. Renninger (Eds.), *Handbook of child psychology* (5th ed., pp. 275–355). New York: Wiley.

Byrne, B., Fielding-Barnsley, R., & Ashley, L. (2000). Effects of preschool phoneme identity training after six years: Outcome level distinguished from rate of response. *Journal of Educational Psychology, 92*(4), 659–667.

Chard, D., & Dickson, S. (1999). Phonological awareness: Instructional and assessment guidelines. *Intervention in School and Clinic, 34*(5), 261–270.

National Reading Panel. (2000). *Report of the National Reading Panel: Reports of the subgroups.* Washington, DC: National Institute of Child Health and Human Development Clearinghouse.

Ochs, K. (2001). *Phonemic awareness: One approach to individualized instruction.* Unpublished specialist's thesis, Eastern Illinois University, Charleston.

Torgesen, J. [K.] (2000). Individual differences in response to early interventions in reading: The lingering problem of treatment resisters. *Learning Disabilities and Practices, 15*, 55–64.

Torgesen, J. K. & Bryant, B. (1994). *Test of Phonological Awareness.* Austin, TX: PRO-ED.

Torgesen, J. K., & Mathes, P. G. (2000). *A basic guide to understanding, assessing, and teaching phonological awareness.* Austin, TX: PRO-ED.

Torgesen, J. [K.], Wagner, R., Rashotte, C., Rose, E., Lindamood, P. Conway, T., & Garvan, C. (1999). Preventing reading failure in young children with phonological processing disabilities: Group and individual responses to instruction. *Journal of Educational Psychology, 91*(4), 579–593.

Assessment for Individualized Lessons

Name _____ Date _____

Pre _____ Post _____

INITIAL SOUNDS

Directions: "I am going to say a word, and I want you to say the first sound in that word. Let me show you. If I say 'mouse,' you would say /mmm/; /mmm/ is the first sound in mouse. Now here's one for you: 'move.' Say the first sound in 'move.'" If the child does not say /mmm/, say "/mmm/ is the first sound in move. Listen: mmmove. Now you tell me the first sound in each word I say."

Scoring: One point for each first sound produced in isolation; 6 points are possible.

Score 0/1		Child's Response	Score 0/1		Child's Response
1. ____	"sand"	_____	4. ____	"nice"	_____
2. ____	"farm"	_____	5. ____	"mud"	_____
3. ____	"pet"	_____	6. ____	"tub"	_____

Score for 1–6: ____ / 6

FINAL SOUNDS

Directions: "Now I am going to say a word and I want you so say the *last* sound in that word. Let me show you. If I say 'cat,' you would say /t/; /t/ is the last sound in 'cat.' Now you do this one: 'night.' Say the <u>last</u> sound in 'night.'" If the child does not say /t/, say "The last sound in night is /t/. Listen: nigh/t/, /t/. Now tell me the <u>last</u> sound in each word I say."

Scoring: One point for each last sound produced in isolation; 6 points are possible.

Score 0/1		Child's Response	Score 0/1		Child's Response
7. ____	"lap"	_____	10. ____	"home"	_____
8. ____	"win"	_____	11. ____	"leaf"	_____
9. ____	"shirt"	_____	12. ____	"goose"	_____

Score for 7–12: ____ / 6

SOUND–LETTER SPELLING

Directions: After you place the letters (*m, s, f, n, p, t, a, i*) in random order on the table, say "You choose from these letters to make each word that I say. Make the word as best you can. Put the letters for each word right here." Mix and replace the letters above the child's work space after each response.

Scoring: One point for each correct first and/or last letter; ignore any extra letters between the first and last letters; 12 points are possible.

Score 0–2	Child's Response	Score 0–2	Child's Response
13. ____ "tan" _____		16. ____ "pat" _____	
14. ____ "sip" _____		17. ____ "nip" _____	
15. ____ "fit" _____		18. ____ "mit" _____	

Score for 13–18: ____ / 12

TOTAL SCORE: ____ / 24

Letters for Assessment Measure

m	s	f
a	i	
n	p	t

Progress Chart

Lessons

Child's name	Preassessment (from Chapter 4) Date	Beginning sounds /m/, /s/ 1	Beginning sounds /f/, /n/ 2	Beginning sounds /p/, /t/ 3	Beginning sounds review 4	Beginning letters m, s 5	Beginning letters f, n 6	Beginning letters p, t 7	Beginning letters m, s, f 8	Beginning letters n, p, t 9	Beginning letters review 10	Ending letters n, p, t 11	Ending sounds /n/, /p/, /t/ 12	Ending sounds /n/, /p/, /t/ 13	Beginning m, s, f Ending n, p, t 14	Beginning n, p, t Ending n, p, t 15	Beginning and ending 16	Tiny books	Postassessment (from Chapter 4) Date

Chapter 5

The Individualized Lessons

Lesson 1: Beginning Sounds /m/ and /s/

Preparation

1. Copy and cut the page of teacher's pictures for Lesson 1.
2. Copy and cut the page of child's pictures for Lesson 1 for each child.
3. Copy the Activity Page (Lesson 1) for each child.

Procedure

Begin the lessons by saying to the child, "I am going to help you during these lessons to learn more about sounds and letters. This will help you when you learn to read."

1. With the stack of /m/ pictures in hand, say, "The words for these pictures begin with /mmm/. Listen: /mmm/onkey." Lay down the monkey picture. Name each picture, emphasizing /mmm/ as you lay it in a column beneath the monkey picture.
2. With the stack of /s/ pictures in hand, say, "The words for these pictures begin with /sss/. Listen: /sss/nake." Lay the snake picture down well to the right of the monkey picture. Name each picture emphasizing the /sss/ as you lay it in a column under the snake picture.
3. Teacher: "Now you say the word for each picture that begins with /m/." Point to each picture, and have the child say the word. If the initial sound is not clear, model saying the word while the child watches your mouth and ask the child to say the word again.
4. Continue: "Now you say the word for each picture that begins with /s/." Point to each picture, and have the child say the word. If the initial sound is not clear, model saying the word while the child watches your mouth and ask the child to say the word again.
5. Pick up the pictures under the monkey and snake and mix them. Give the stack of pictures to the child: "Now it's your turn to say the word for each picture and put it under the monkey if it begins with /m/ or under the snake if it begins with /s/." If the child has difficulty, model the correct response by saying the word while emphasizing the initial sound and place it in the correct column. If a child does not readily name the picture or labels it as something else, remove that picture from the lesson for that child.
6. Give the child the Activity Page with the monkey and snake at the top. Mix the child's six pictures for this activity and give them one at a time to the child: "Tell me the word for this picture, and then tape [glue] it under the monkey if that picture begins with /m/ or under the snake if it begins with /s/." If the child begins to place a picture incorrectly, ask him or her to repeat the name of the picture and help the child to correctly place it.
7. After the six pictures are correctly in place, ask the child to name each of the pictures that begins with /m/ and then each that begins with /s/. Say, "You can take this page home and tell your family (or mom or dad) that you know some words that start with /m/ and /s/."
8. At the completion of the lesson, allow the child to choose one from several stickers and check the Progress Chart (at the end of Chapter 4) for Lesson 1.

Teacher's Pictures for /m/ (Lesson 1)

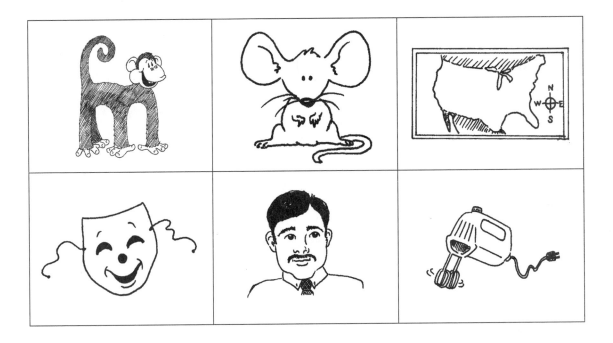

Teacher's Pictures for /s/ (Lesson 1)

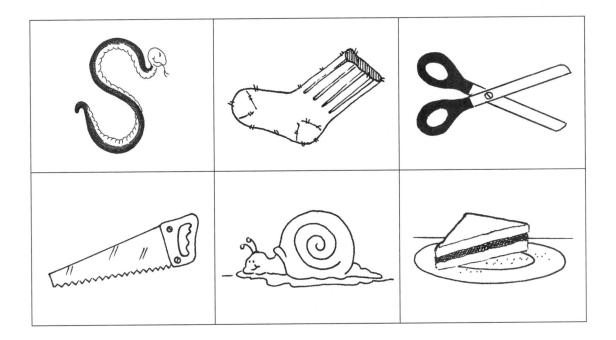

Child's Activity Page Pictures for /m/ (Lesson 1)

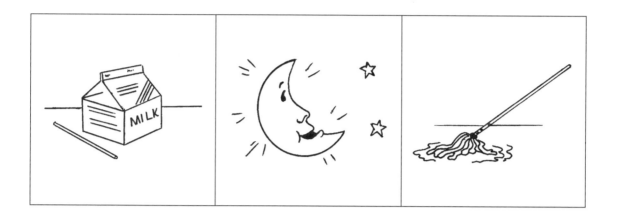

Child's Activity Page Pictures for /s/ (Lesson 1)

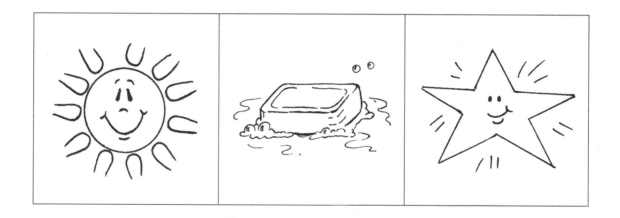

Activity Page (Lesson 1)

Name _____

Beginning Sound /m/   *Beginning Sound /s/*

   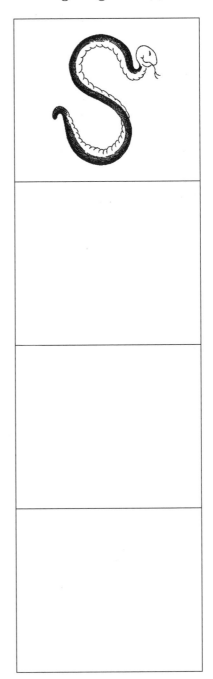

Lesson 2: Beginning Sounds /f/ and /n/

Preparation

1. Copy and cut the page of teacher's pictures for Lesson 2.
2. Copy and cut the page of child's pictures for Lesson 2 for each child.
3. Copy Activity Page 2 for each child.

Procedure

1. Begin with a brief review of /m/ and /s/ at the beginning of words. Say, "Let's see if we can remember words that begin with /m/." Name several words, such as "milk, monster, middle" and ask the child to produce another that begins with /m/. Repeat for /s/, naming several words such as "soap, scissors, silly." If the child cannot generate as least one or two words, repeat Lesson 1.
2. With the stack of /f/ pictures in hand, say, "Now let's practice listening for /fff/ at the beginning of words. Listen: /fff/lower." Lay down the flower picture. Name each picture emphasizing the /fff/ as you lay in it in a column under the flower.
3. With the stack of /n/ pictures in hand, say, "The words for these pictures begin with /nnn/. Listen: /nnn/est." Lay down the nest picture in a column to the right of the flower. Name each picture beginning with /n/ in a column under the nest.
4. Continue: "Now you say the word for each picture that begins with /f/." Point to each picture and have the child say the word. If the initial sound is not clear, model saying the word while the child watches your mouth and ask the child to say the word again.
5. Repeat step 4 for /n/ pictures.
6. Pick up the pictures under the flower and nest, mix them, and give the stack of pictures to the child: "Now it's your turn to say the word for each picture and put it under the flower if it begins with /f/ or under the nest if it begins with /n/." If the child has difficulty, model the correct response by saying the word while emphasizing the initial sound and place it in the correct column. If a child does not readily name the picture, remove that picture from the lesson for that child.
7. Give the child the Activity Page with the flower and nest on the top. Mix the child's six pictures for this activity and give them one at a time to the child. Say, "Tell me the word for this picture and then tape [glue] it under the flower if that picture begins with /f/ or under the nest if it begins with /n/." If the child begins to place a picture incorrectly, ask him or her to repeat the name of the picture and help the child to correctly place it.
8. After the six pictures are correctly in place, ask the child to name the pictures that begin with /f/ and then those that begin with /n/. Tell the child that he or she can take this page home.
9. At the completion of the lesson, allow the child to choose a sticker and check the Progress Chart for Lesson 2.

Teacher's Pictures for /f/ (Lesson 2)

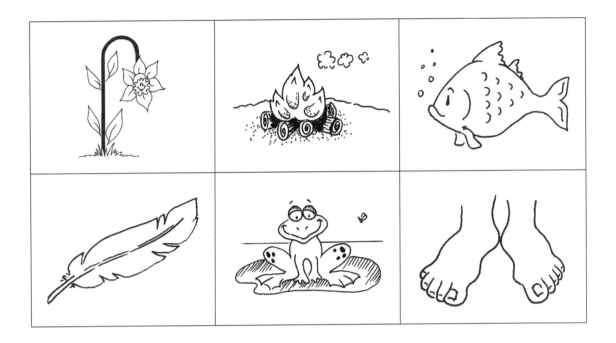

Teacher's Pictures for /n/ (Lesson 2)

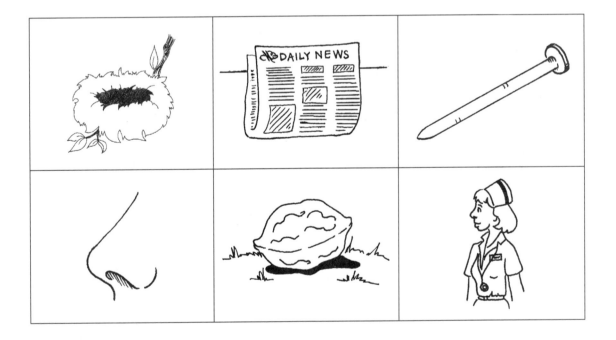

Child's Activity Page Pictures for /f/ (Lesson 2)

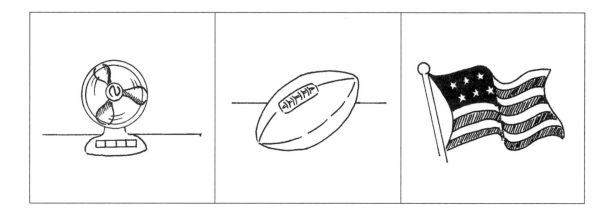

Child's Activity Page Pictures for /n/ (Lesson 2)

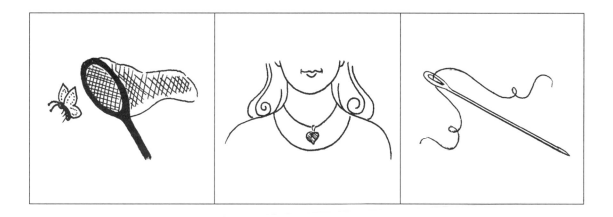

Activity Page (Lesson 2)

Name _____

Beginning Sound /f/	*Beginning Sound /n/*

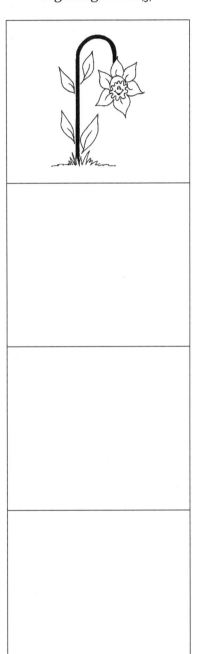

Lesson 3: Beginning Sounds /p/ and /t/

Preparation

1. Copy and cut the page of teacher's pictures for Lesson 3.
2. Copy and cut the page of child's pictures for Lesson 3 for each child.
3. Copy the Activity Page (Lesson 3) for each child.

Procedure

1. Begin with a brief review of /f/ and /n/ at the beginning of words: "Let's see if we can remember words that begin with /f/." Name several words such as "fun, fish, Friday" and ask the child to say another that begins with /f/. If the child cannot think of any words, provide a choice by saying one word that begins with /f/ and a second word that begins with a different consonant. Ask the child which word begins with /f/. Continue with several more examples of two words, asking the child to repeat the word that begins with /f/.

2. Repeat the above procedure for /n/, naming several words such as "nut, nice, noon." Provide a choice of two words as above (one beginning with /n/) if the child cannot generate any words that begin with /n/.

3. With the stack of /p/ pictures in hand, say, "Today our beginning sounds are /p/ and /t/. Let's begin with /p/. Listen: /p/enguin." Lay down the penguin picture. Name each picture beginning with /p/ as you lay in it in a column under the penguin.

4. With the stack of /t/ pictures in hand, say "The words for these pictures begin with /t/. Listen: /t/urtle." Lay down the turtle picture to the right of the penguin. Name each picture beginning with /t/, and lay it in a column under the turtle.

5. Proceed: "Now you say the word for each picture beginning with /p/." Point to each picture under the penguin and have the child say the word that names it. Continue with pictures beginning with /t/. If the initial sound is not clear, model saying the word while the child watches your mouth and ask the child to say the word again.

6. After picking up all the pictures under the penguin and turtle, mix them and give the stack to the child: "Now you say the word for each picture and put it under the penguin if it begins with /p/ or under the turtle if it begins with /t/." If the child has difficulty, model the correct response by saying the word while emphasizing the initial sound, and place it in the correct column. If a child does not readily name the picture, remove that picture from the lesson for that child.

7. Give the child the Activity Page with the penguin and turtle on the top. Mix the child's six pictures for this activity, and give them one at a time to the child. Say, "Tell me the word for this picture and then tape [glue] it under the penguin if the word begins with /p/ or under the turtle if it begins with /t/." If the child begins to place a picture incorrectly, ask him or her to repeat the name of the picture and check if it begins with /p/ or /t/.

8. After the six pictures are correctly in place, ask the child to name the pictures that begin with /p/ and then those that begin with /t/. Tell the child that he or she can take this page home.

9. At the completion of the lesson, allow the child to choose a sticker and check the Progress Chart for Lesson 3.

Teacher's Pictures for /p/ (Lesson 3)

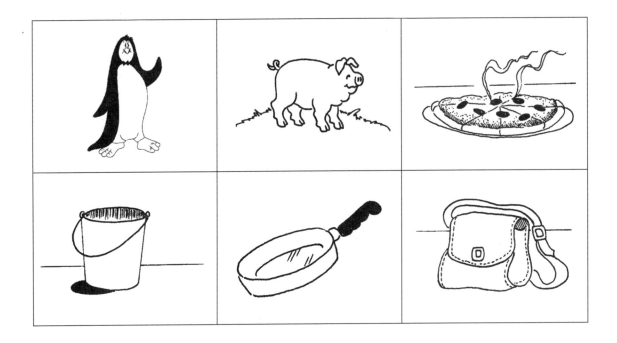

Teacher's Pictures for /t/ (Lesson 3)

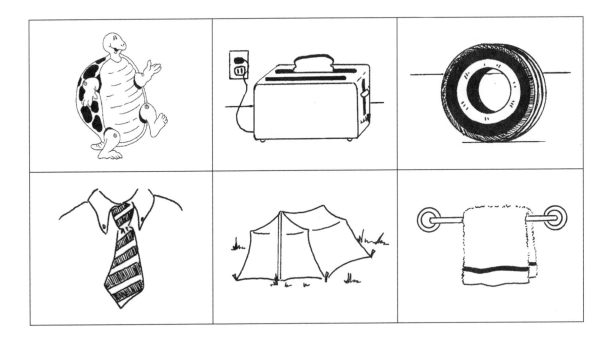

Child's Activity Page Pictures for /p/ (Lesson 3)

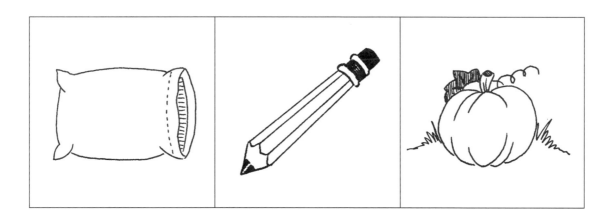

Child's Activity Page Pictures for /t/ (Lesson 3)

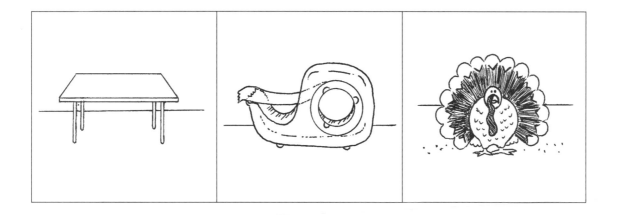

Activity Page (Lesson 3)

Name _____

Beginning Sound /p/	*Beginning Sound /t/*

Lesson 4: Review of Beginning Sounds

Preparation

1. Assemble all teacher's pictures for beginning sounds from previous lessons in a separate stack for each beginning sound.

Procedure

1. Place the monkey, snake, and flower pictures in a row across the top of your work space. Mix the remaining pictures for these three sounds.
2. Teacher: "Let's practice our beginning sounds. I will give you one picture at a time. You tell me the word for that picture, and then put it under the picture that has the same beginning sound."
3. Give the child one picture at a time. If the child does not correctly label the picture, remove it from the lesson for that child. After all the pictures have been placed, pick up the pictures for each beginning sound in a separate stack.
4. Place the nest, turtle, and penguin pictures in a row across the top of your work space. Mix the remaining pictures for these three sounds.
5. Teacher: "Let's practice these beginning sounds. I will give you one picture at a time. You tell me the word for that picture, and then put it under the picture that has the same beginning sound."
6. Give the child one picture at a time. If the child does not correctly label a picture, remove it from the lesson for that child. After all the pictures have been placed, pick up the pictures for each beginning sound in a separate stack.
7. Repeat the procedure in steps 1 to 3, above, with all six beginning sounds. If the child has difficulty, repeat lessons for which beginning sounds cannot be identified.
8. At the completion of the lesson, allow the child to choose a sticker and check the Progress Chart for Lesson 4.

Lesson 5: Letters *m* and *s* for Beginning Sounds

Preparation

1. Copy and cut the page of teacher's pictures for Lesson 5.
2. Copy and cut the page of child's pictures for Lesson 5 for each child.
3. Copy the Activity Page (Lesson 5) for each child.

Procedure

1. Place the monkey picture with the embedded *m* and the letter *m* square underneath it in front of the child as you say, "The letter *m* stands for the /mmm/ sound. The letter *m* in the monkey picture can help you remember that *m* stands for the sound /m/." Point out the letter *m* in the monkey picture.
2. Place the snake picture with the embedded *s* and the letter *s* square underneath it in front of the child as you say, "The letter *s* stands for the /sss/ sound. The *s* in the snake picture can help you remember that *s* stands for the sound /s/." Point out the *s* in the snake picture.
3. Say the word for each of the accompanying four pictures for *m* and place under the monkey and *m*. Then say the words for each of the four pictures for *s* and place under the snake and *s*.
4. Pick up all the pictures but not the letters *m* and *s*. Say, "Point to the letter for /mmm/; point to the letter for /sss/." If the child has difficulty, place the monkey under the *m* and say, "*m* stands for the /mmm/ in monkey'"; place the snake under the *s* and say, "*s* stands for the /sss/ in 'snake.'" Leave the monkey and snake in place.
5. Mix the pictures and give them one at a time to the child. Say, "Tell me the word for this picture, and put it under the *m* if it begins with /m/ or under the *s* if it begins with /s/." If the child begins to make a wrong choice, ask him or her to listen to you say the word. Then ask the child to say the word again and direct him or her to the correct letter if needed.
6. Give the child the Activity Page with *m* and *s* on the top. Mix the child's six pictures for this activity and give them one at a time to the child: "Tell me the word for each picture, and then tape [glue] it under the letter for the beginning sound." If the child begins to place a picture incorrectly, ask him or her to say the word again and then to say just the first sound. Help the child to place it under the correct letter.
7. Tell the child that he or she may take this page home and can show the family that he or she knows words that begin with *s* or *m*.
8. At the completion of the lesson, allow the child to choose a sticker and check the Progress Chart for Lesson 5.

Teacher's Pictures for Letter *m* (Lesson 5)

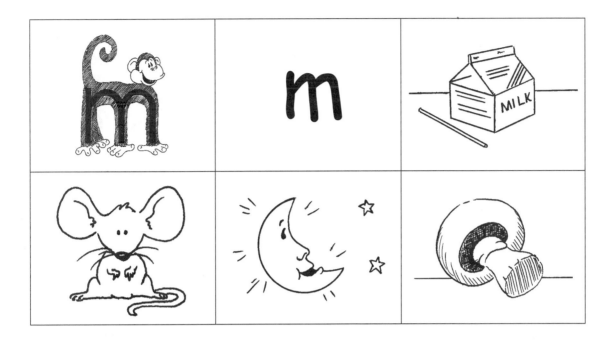

Teacher's Pictures for Letter *s* (Lesson 5)

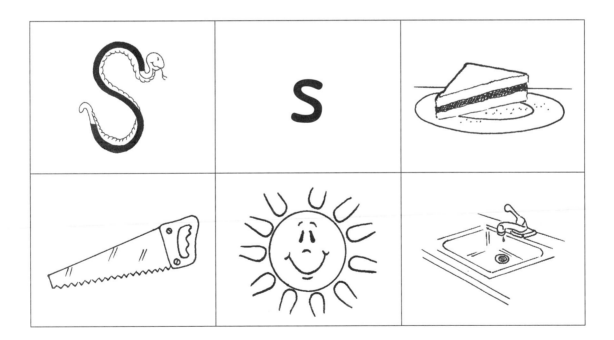

Child's Activity Page Pictures for Letter *m* (Lesson 5)

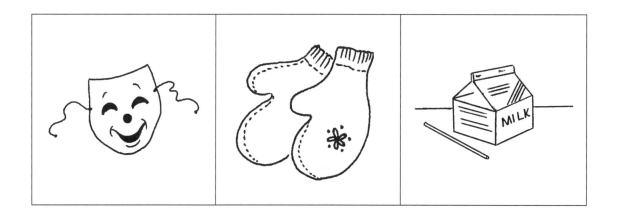

Child's Activity Page Pictures for Letter *s* (Lesson 5)

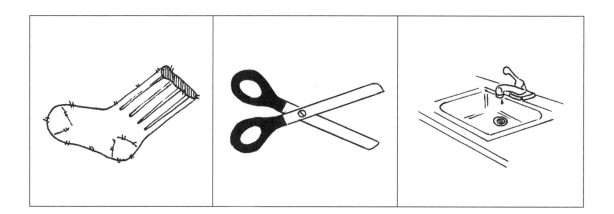

Activity Page (Lesson 5)

Name _____

Beginning Letter m	Beginning Letter s
m	s

Lesson 6: Letters *f* and *n* for Beginning Sounds

Preparation

1. Copy and cut the page of teacher's pictures for Lesson 6.
2. Copy and cut the page of child's pictures for Lesson 6 for each child.
3. Copy the Activity Page (Lesson 6) for each child.

Procedure

1. Teacher: "First let's practice thinking of some words that begin with the letter *m*." Give several examples such as "monkey, milk, mom." Ask the child to think of another word that begins with the letter *m*.
2. Continue: "Now let's practice thinking of some words that begin with the letter *s*." Give several examples such as "snake, sister, summer." Ask the child to think of another word that begins with the letter *s*.
3. Place the flower picture with the embedded *f* and the letter *f* square underneath it in front of the child as you say, "The letter *f* stands for the /fff/ sound. The *f* in the flower picture can help you remember that *f* stands for the sound /fff/." Point to the *f* in the flower picture.
4. Place the nest picture with the embedded *n* and the letter *n* square underneath it in front of the child as you say, "The *n* in the nest picture can help you remember that *n* stands for the sound /n/." Point to the *n* in the nest picture.
5. Say the words depicted by each of the accompanying four pictures for *f*, and place them under the flower. Then say the words depicted by each of the four pictures for *n*, and place them under the nest.
6. Pick up all the pictures but not the letters *f* and *n*. Say, "Point to the letter for /fff/; point to the letter for /nnn/." If the child has difficulty, place the flower under the *f* and say, "*f* stands for the /fff/ in 'flower'"; place the nest under the *n* and say, "*n* stands for the /nnn/ in 'nest.'" Leave the flower and nest pictures in place.
7. Mix the pictures and give them one at a time to the child: "Tell me the word for each picture, and put it under the *f* if it begins with /f/ or under the *n* if it begins with /n/." If the child begins to make a wrong choice, ask him or her to listen to you say the word. Then ask the child to say the word again, and direct him or her to the correct letter if necessary.
8. Give the child the Activity Page with the *f* and *n* on top. Mix the child's six pictures for this activity, and give them one at a time to the child: "Tell me the word for each picture, and then tape [glue] it under the letter that stands for the beginning sound." If the child begins to place a picture incorrectly, ask him or her to say the word again and then to say just the first sound. Help the child place it under the correct letter.
9. At the completion of the lesson, allow the child to choose a sticker and check the Progress Chart for Lesson 6.

Teacher's Pictures for Letter *f* (Lesson 6)

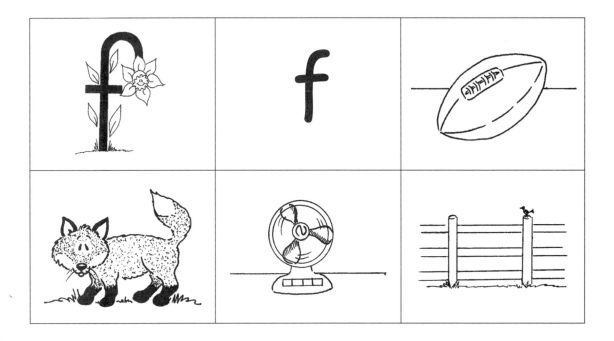

Teacher's Pictures for Letter *n* (Lesson 6)

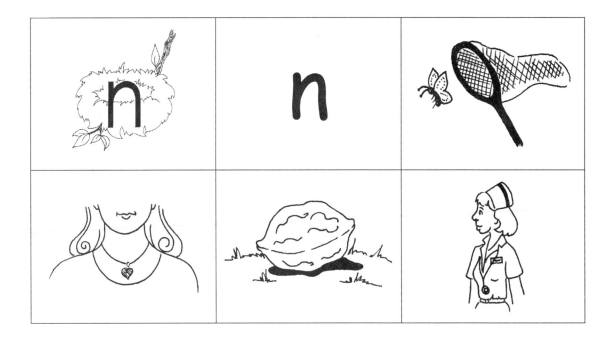

Child's Activity Page Pictures for Letter *f* (Lesson 6)

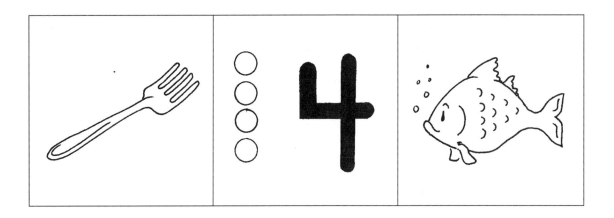

Child's Activity Page Pictures for Letter *n* (Lesson 6)

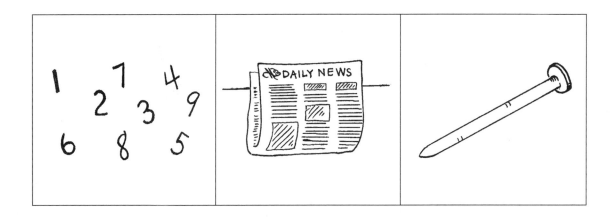

Activity Page (Lesson 6)

Name _____

Beginning Letter f	*Beginning Letter n*
f	n

Lesson 7: Letters *p* and *t* for Beginning Sounds

Preparation

1. Copy and cut the page of teacher's pictures for Lesson 7.
2. Copy and cut the page of child's pictures for Lesson 7 for each child.
3. Copy the Activity Page (Lesson 7) for each child.

Procedure

1. Teacher: "Let's first think of some words that begin with the letter *f* as we practiced last time." Give several examples such as "flower, fun, fire." Ask the child to think of a few more words that begin with *f*.
2. Continue: "Now let's practice thinking of words that begin with the letter *n*. Give several examples such as "nest, no, nine." Ask the child to say some more words that begin with *n*.
3. Place the penguin picture with the embedded *p* and the letter *p* square underneath it in front of the child as you say, "The letter *p* stands for the /p/ sound. The *p* in the penguin picture can help you remember that *p* stands for the sound /p/."
4. Place the turtle picture with the embedded *t* and the letter *t* square underneath it in front of the child as you say "The *t* in the turtle picture can help you remember that *t* stands for the sound /t/."
5. Say the words depicted by each of the accompanying four pictures for *p* and place them under the penguin. Then say the words depicted by each of the four pictures for *t* and place them under the turtle.
6. Pick up all the pictures but not the *p* and *t*. Say, "Point to the letter for /p/; point to the letter for /t/." If the child has difficulty, place the penguin under the *p* and say, "*p* stands for the /p/ in 'penguin'"; place the turtle under the *t* and say, "*t* stands for the /t/ in 'turtle.'" Leave the penguin and turtle pictures in place.
7. Mix the pictures, and give them one at a time to the child. Say, "Tell me the word for each picture, and put it under the *p* if it begins with /p/ or under the *t* if it begins with /t/." If the child begins to make a wrong choice, ask him or her to listen to you say the word. Then ask the child to say the word again and direct him or her to the correct letter if necessary.
8. Give the child the Activity Page with *p* and *t* on the top. Mix the child's six pictures for this activity, and give them one at a time to the child: "Tell me the word for each picture, and then tape [glue] it under the letters *p* or *t*." If the child begins to place a picture incorrectly, ask him or her to say the word again and then to say just the first sound. Help the child to place it under the correct letter.
9. At the completion of the lesson, allow the child to choose a sticker and check the Progress Chart for Lesson 7.

Teacher's Pictures for Letter *p* (Lesson 7)

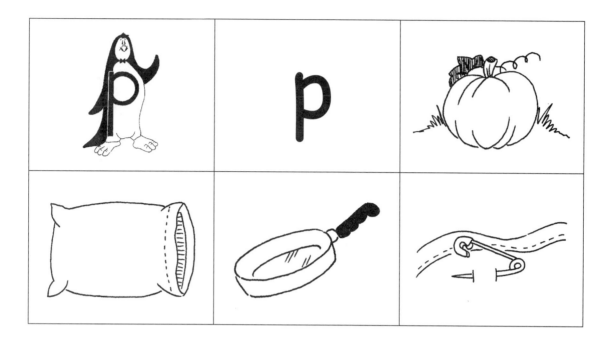

Teacher's Pictures for Letter *t* (Lesson 7)

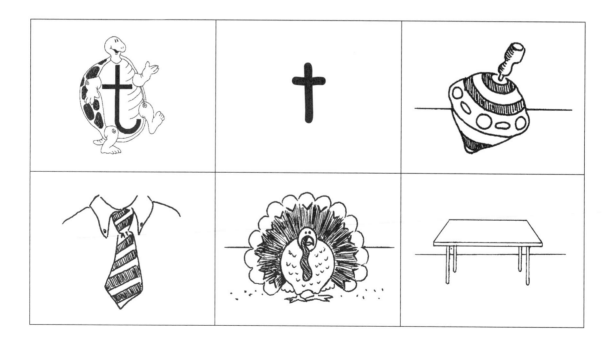

Child's Activity Page Pictures for Letter *p* (Lesson 7)

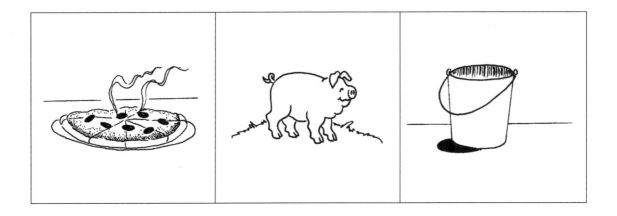

Child's Activity Page Pictures for Letter *t* (Lesson 7)

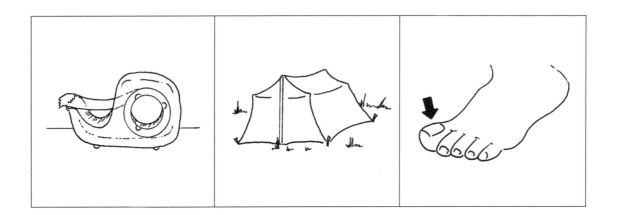

Activity Page (Lesson 7)

Name _____

Beginning Letter p	Beginning Letter t
p	t

Lesson 8: Letters *m*, *s*, and *f* for Beginning Sounds

Preparation

1. Copy and cut the teacher's page (including blank squares) for Lesson 8.
2. Copy and cut the child's letter squares page and the Activity Page (Lesson 8) for each child.

Procedure

1. Place the letter squares for *m*, *s*, and *f* at the top of the work space and the six blank squares to the right of the letter squares.
2. Lay out in a column beneath the letter squares the pictures for "sit," "man," and "fin."
3. Teacher: "Today, we are going to use these letters (*point to letters*) for the first sound in each of these words."
4. Continue: "Let's begin with 'sit': /sss/it. The first sound in 'sit' is /sss/, so I'll use the *s* for /sss/." Pick up the letter *s* and place it to the right of the picture for "sit." "I'll use these blank squares for the other sounds in 'sit.' Here's the *s* for /sss/ (*point to the s*), and then I'll put this (*a blank square*) for the /i/ and another for /t/." Lay the blank squares to the right of the *s*.
5. Follow the same procedure in step 4 with the pictures for "man" and "fin."
6. Pick up the pictures, letter squares, and blank squares.
7. Place the child's letter squares at the top of the work space and give the child the Activity Page with the pictures for "sun," "fan," and "map." Say, "Now it is your turn to pick the letter for the first sound in each of these words."
8. Continue: "Tell me the word for this picture (*point to the sun*). For now we are just choosing the letter for the first sound, so you choose the letter for /sss/ and put it here" as you point to the first line to the right of the sun. After the child places the *s* on the first line, say, "Here is the *s* for /sss/, this space is for the /u/, and this for the /n/" as you point to the second and third lines. "Now you tape [glue] the letter *s* in place as the beginning sound in 'sun.'" The child can tape [glue] blank squares for the last two sounds if he or she is interested in doing so.
9. Repeat the same procedure in step 8 with the fan and map.
10. After all three pictures are completed, say, "Point to the letter for /sss/ in 'sun.'" After the child points to the *s*, say, "Now point to the letter for the /fff/ in 'fan.'" After the child points to the *f*, continue with the /mmm/ in "map." Then tell the child that he or she may take this page home and show it to the family.
11. At the completion of the lesson, allow the child to choose a sticker and check the Progress Chart for Lesson 8.

Teacher's Pictures and Letters *m*, *s*, and *f* for Beginning Sounds
(Lesson 8)

m	s	f

Child's Letters: *m*, *s*, and *f* for Beginning Sounds (Lesson 8)

m	s	f

Activity Page (Lesson 8)

Name _____

Beginning Letters m, s, f

_____ _____ _____

_____ _____ _____

_____ _____ _____

Lesson 9: Letters *n*, *p*, and *t* for Beginning Sounds

Preparation

1. Copy and cut the teacher's page (including blank squares) for Lesson 9.
2. Copy and cut the child's letter squares page and the Activity Page (Lesson 9) for each child.

Procedure

1. Place the letter squares for *n*, *p*, and *t* at the top of the work space; put the blank squares to the right of the letters.
2. Lay out in a column the pictures for "top," "pan," and "nut."
3. Teacher: "Today, we are going to use these letters (*point to letters*) for the first sound in each of these words."
4. Continue: "Let's begin with 'top.': /t/op. The first sound in 'top' is /t/, so I'll use the *t* for /t/." Pick up the letter *t* and place it to the right of the picture. "I'll use these blank squares for the other sounds in 'top.' Here's the *t* for /t/; then I'll put this (*point to a blank square*) for the /o/ and another for the /p/." Lay the blank squares to the left of the *t*.
5. Follow the same procedure in step 4 with the pictures for "pan" and "nut."
6. Pick up the pictures, letters, and blank squares.
7. Place the child's letter squares at the top of the work space and give the child the Activity Page with the pictures for "pin," "ten," and "net." Say, "Now it is your turn to pick the letter for the first sound in each of these words."
8. Proceed: "Tell me the word for this picture" (*point to the pin*). For now we are choosing just the letter for the first sound, so you choose the letter for /p/ and put it right here" (*point to the first line to the right of the pin*). After the child places the *p* on the first line, say, "Here is the *p* for /p/, this space is for the /i/, and this for the /n/ (*point to the blank lines*). Now you tape [glue] the letter *p* in place as the beginning sound in 'pin.'"
9. Repeat the procedure in step 8 with the pictures for "ten" and "net."
10. After all three beginning letters are chosen, say, "Point to the letter for /p/ in 'pin.'" After the child points to the *p*, say, "Now point to the /t/ in 'ten.'" After the child points to the *t*, continue with the /n/ in "net." Tell the child that he or she may take this page home.
11. At the completion of the lesson, allow the child to choose a sticker and check the Progress Chart for Lesson 9.

Teacher's Pictures and Letters *n*, *p*, and *t* for Beginning Sounds (Lesson 9)

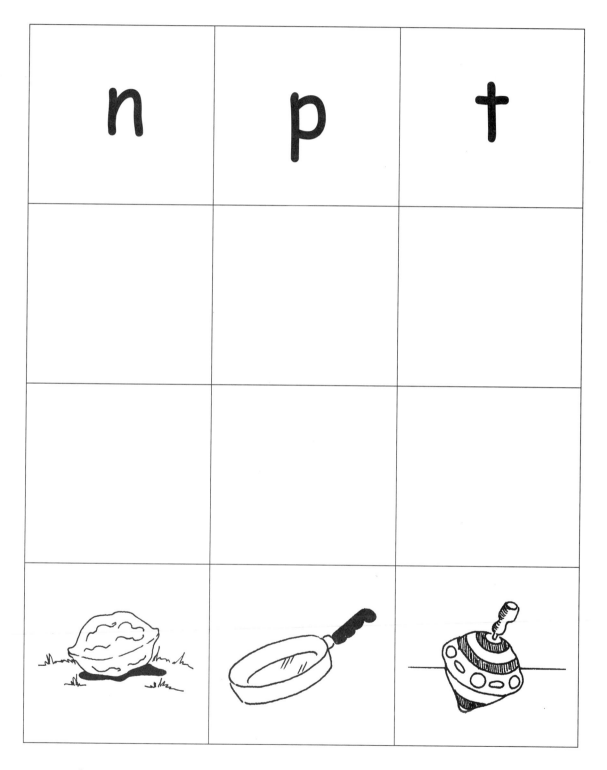

Child's Letters: *n*, *p*, and *t* for Beginning Sounds (Lesson 9)

n	p	t

Activity Page (Lesson 9)

Name _____

Beginning Letters n, p, t

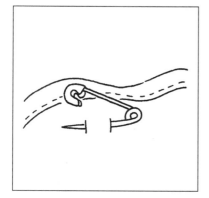

_____ _____ _____

10

_____ _____ _____

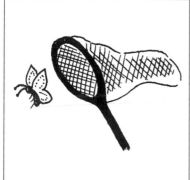

_____ _____ _____

Lesson 10: Review of Letters for Beginning Sounds

Preparation

1. Copy and cut the teacher's page for Lesson 10.

Procedure

1. Lay the letter squares for *m*, *s*, *f*, *n*, *p*, and *t* at the top of the work space.
2. Teacher: "Today let's practice choosing the first letter in words without pictures. After I say a word, you give me the letter for the first sound in that word." Replace the letter on the table after the child makes his or her choice. If the child is unsure or chooses an incorrect letter, say, "Let's do that word again. Listen when I say it again." Repeat the word, emphasizing the first sound. "Now you say the word before you choose the letter for the first sound." If the child continues to have difficulty, ask the child to repeat the first sound and then point out the letter that matches this sound.
3. Use the following words, or choose words that you think the child knows well:

   monkey, mom, snake, sis, mountain, scissors, sandwich, muscle

   sun, flower, mat, nest, fun, night, mushroom, fish

   turtle, penguin, turkey, pill, mittens, sink, flag, nose

   met, fit, nap, sit, tip, pat, pot, tin

4. If at any point the child loses interest in the lesson, stop shortly thereafter. If this is because the child is sure of the beginning sounds and letters, go on to the next lesson. If this is because the child is unsure of any of the beginning sounds, give a few more examples beginning with words you think the child may know. Note the difficult sounds, and begin the next lesson with a review of these beginning sounds.
5. At the completion of the lesson, allow the child to choose a sticker and check the Progress Chart for Lesson 10.

Teacher's Letters for Beginning Sounds Review (Lesson 10)

m	s	f
n	p	t

Lesson 11: Letters *n*, *p*, *t* for Ending Sounds

Preparation

1. Copy and cut teacher's page for Lesson 11.
2. Copy the child's page of letter squares and the Activity Page (Lesson 11) for each child.

Procedure

1. Teacher: "Today we are going to listen for the *ending* or *last* sound in words. This is new and can be hard, but it will help you when you learn to read. Let's practice together."
2. Lay out the *n*, *p*, and *t* letter squares in a row and the pictures of the sun, the mop, and the nut in a column under the first letter square. Put the blank squares in a stack to the right of the letter squares.
3. Begin with the word "sun": "Let's listen for the last sound in the word 'sun,' /s/, /u/, /n/. The last sound is /n/." Say the word again slowly as you place blank squares in a row to the right of the sun for first two sounds and the *n* letter square for the last sound. Say "sun" again as you point to the corresponding square for each sound.
4. Repeat the procedure in step 3 with the pictures for "mop" and "nut."
5. Pick up the letter and blank squares and place the letter squares in a row at the top of the work space. Then pick up the pictures, and lay the mop picture on the table. Say, "Now it's your turn. Listen as I say the word: /m/ /o/ /p/. I'll put this for the /m/ (*place a blank square to the right of the picture*) and this for the /o/ (*place a blank square next in line*); /p/ is the ending sound in 'mop.' You choose the letter for /p/ and put it here (*point to the right of the blank squares*). If the child has difficulty, repeat "mop" and say, "/p/ is the ending sound in 'mop.' Find the letter for /p/."
6. Repeat the procedure in step 6 with the pictures for "sun" and "nut."
7. Place the child's letter squares at the top of the work space and give the child the Activity Page with the pictures for "top," "pan," and "mat." Say, "Now you can do the ending sound in these words. Let's start with 'top.' I'll put this (*place a blank square*) for the /t/, this for the /o/ (*place a blank square*), and you pick the letter for /p/." If the child has difficulty, repeat the /p/ and ask which letter stands for /p/. After the child has selected the *p*, ask him or her to tape [glue] it on the last line next to the picture of the top.
8. Repeat the procedure in step 7 with the pictures for "pan" and "mat." When the last sound for all three words have been placed, ask the child to say each word and then repeat the last sound in that word. Point out the letter for each last sound.
9. At the completion of the lesson, allow the child to choose a sticker and check the Progress Chart for Lesson 11.

Note: Ending sounds can be much more difficult than beginning sounds, so progressing through these lessons may be slow and require corrective help.

Teacher's Pictures and Letters: *n*, *p*, and *t* for Ending Sounds (Lesson 11)

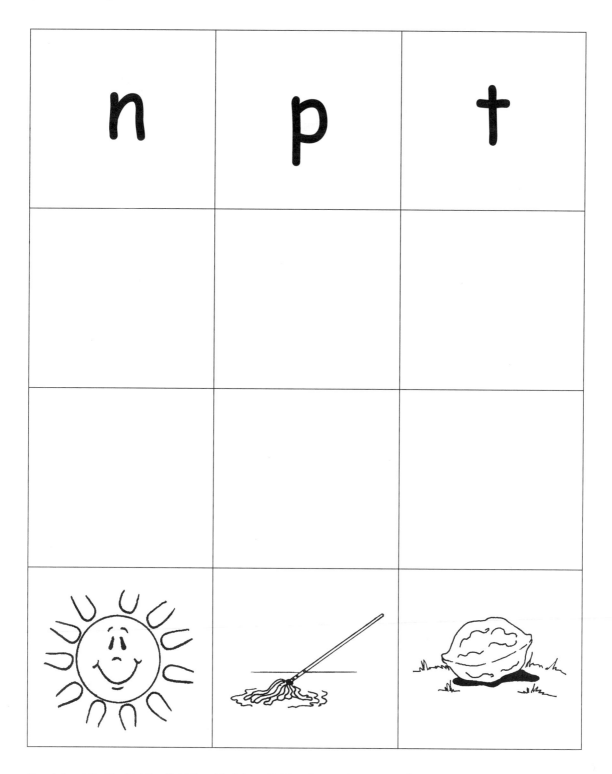

Child's Letters: *n*, *p*, and *t* for Ending Sounds (Lesson 11)

n	p	t

Activity Page (Lesson 11)

Name _____

Beginning Letters n, p, t

_____   _____   _____

_____   _____   _____

Welcome

_____   _____   _____

Lesson 12: Ending Sounds /n/, /p/, and /t/

Preparation

1. Copy and cut teacher's pictures 1 for Lesson 12.

Procedure

1. Begin with teacher's pictures 1. With the stack of pictures ending in /n/ in hand, say, "The words for these pictures end with /nnn/. Listen: ma/nnn/" (*lay down the picture of the man*)." Name each picture, emphasizing the /nnn/ as you lay in it in a column beneath the picture of a man.
2. Teacher: "Now you say the word for each picture that ends with /n/." Point to each picture, and have the child say the word. If the child does not clearly say the ending sound, you say the word and ask him or her to repeat the last sound. Then ask the child to repeat the entire word.
3. With the stack of pictures ending in /p/ in hand, say, "The words for these pictures end with /p/. Listen: ma/p/." Name each picture ending with /p/, and place it in a column under the map.
4. Continue: "Now you say the word for each picture that ends with /p/." Point to each picture and have the child say the word. If the child does not clearly say the ending sound, you say the word and ask him or her to repeat the last sound. Then ask the child to repeat the entire word.
5. With the stack of pictures ending with /t/ in hand, say, "The words for these pictures end with /t/. Listen: ma/t/." Name each picture ending with /t/, and place it in a column under the mat.
6. Proceed: "Now you say the word for each picture that ends with /t/." Point to each picture and have the child say the word. If the child does not clearly say the ending sound, you say the word and ask him or her to repeat the last sounds. Then ask the child to repeat the entire word.
7. Pick up the pictures—except those of the man, the map, and the mat—and mix them. Give the stack of pictures to the child and say, "Name each picture, and put it under the man if it ends with /n/, under the map if it ends with /p/, or under the mat if it ends with /t/," pointing to each picture as you name it. If the child has difficulty, model the correct response by saying the word while emphasizing the ending sound and place it in the correct column. If a child does not readily name the picture, remove that picture from the lesson for that child.
8. At the completion of the lesson, allow the child to choose a sticker and check the Progress Chart for Lesson 12.

Note: If the child is having difficulty identifying the ending sound in the words in this lesson, repeat the lesson next session using the pictures from teacher's page 2.

Teacher's Pictures 1: Ending Sounds /n/, /p/, and /t/ (Lesson 12)

/n/ /p/ /t/

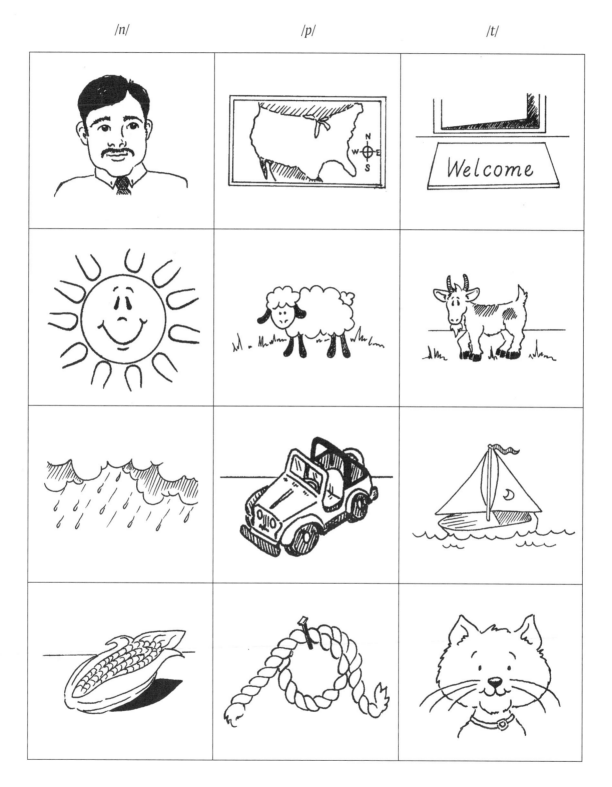

Teacher's Pictures 2: Ending Sounds /n/, /p/, and /t/ (Lesson 12)

| /n/ | /p/ | /t/ |

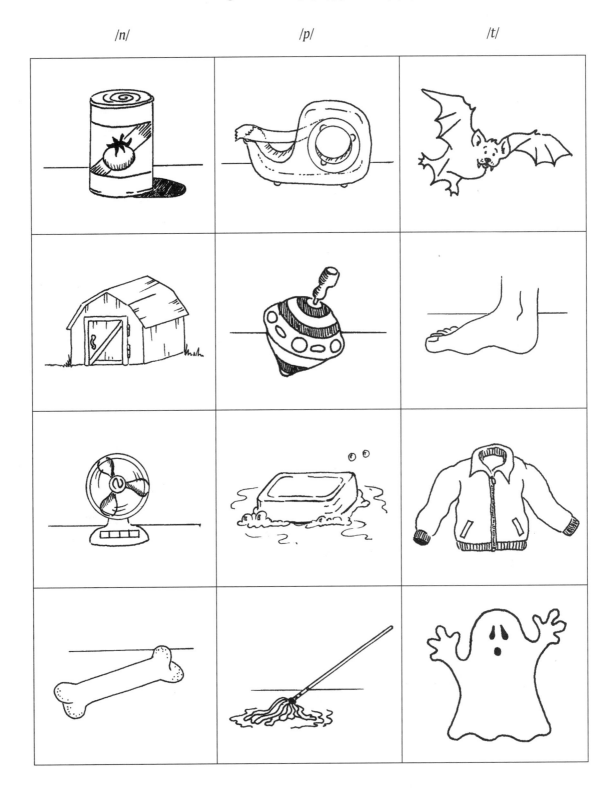

Lesson 13: Ending Sounds /n/, /p/, and /t/

Preparation

1. Copy and cut child's pictures page for each child.
2. Copy and cut the Activity Page (Lesson 13) for each child.

Procedure

1. Give the child the Activity Page with the man, map, and mat on the top of the page. Say, "To-day we are going to listen for the ending or last sound in words again. The ending sound in 'man' is /nnn/, the ending sound in 'map' is /p/, and the ending sound in 'mat' is /t/ (*pointing to each picture as you say the word*). Now you tell me the ending sound in 'man.'" After the child says /n/, proceed to ask about the ending sounds in "map" and "mat."
2. Continue: "Now it is your turn to listen for the last sounds in the words." After mixing the nine pictures for this activity, give them one at a time to the child and say, "Tell me the word for this picture." After the child tells you the word, say, "Now tell me just the last sound." After the child repeats the ending sound correctly, ask him or her to tape [glue] it under the picture of the "man" if that word ends with /n/, under the illustration of a "map" if that word ends with /p/, or under the drawing of a "mat" if that word ends with /t/. If the child begins to place a picture incorrectly, ask him or her to repeat the name of the picture and check if it ends with /n/, /p/ or /t/.
3. After the nine pictures are correctly in place, ask the child to name the pictures ending with /n/, then those ending with /p/, and then those ending with /t/.
4. At the completion of the lesson, allow the child to choose a sticker and check the Progress Chart for Lesson 13.

Child's Pictures: Ending Sounds /n/, /p/, and /t/ (Lesson 13)

/n/   /p/   /t/

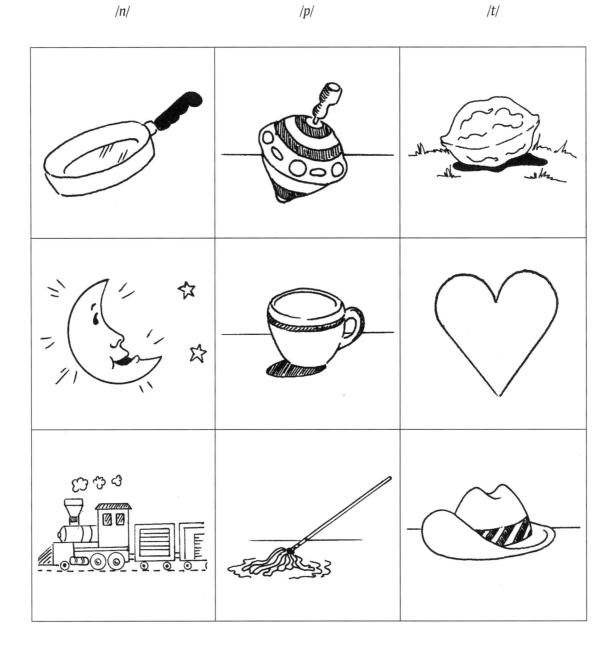

Activity Page (Lesson 13)

Name _____

Ending Sounds n, p, t

		Welcome

Lesson 14: Beginning Letters *m*, *s*, *f* and Ending Letters *n*, *p*, *t*

Preparation

1. Copy and cut teacher's page for Lesson 14.
2. Copy and cut child's page of letter squares and the Activity Page (Lesson 14) for each child.

Procedure

1. Place the teacher's letter and blank squares at the top of the work space.
2. Lay out in a column beneath the letters the pictures of the mop, the fat (person), and the sun.
3. Teacher: "Today we are going to use these letters for the beginning *and* ending sounds in the words for these pictures. Let's begin with 'mop.'"
4. Continue: "The first sound in 'mop' is /m/, so I'll put *m* here (*to the right of the pictured mop*). Next I'll put this (*a blank square*) for the /o/ and then *p* for the /p/." Say "mop" slowly, and point to each square as you say the sound.
5. Repeat the procedure in step 4 with the pictures of the fat (person) and the sun.
6. Remove the letter and blank squares and replace them at the top of the work space. Say, "Now you do the first and last sounds for each of the words just as I did."
7. Pointing to the mop, say, "Tell me the word for this picture. . . . Right. Now tell me just the first sound." After the child replies with the sound /m/, say, "Now pick the letter for /m/ and place it here" as you point to the right of the picture. Say, "I'll put this (*a blank square*) for the /o/ and you pick the letter for /p/ and put it here (*point to the right of the blank square*)." "Let's check: /m/ (*point to the m*), /o/ (*point to the blank*), /p/ (*point to the p*)—'mop.'"
8. Repeat the procedure in step 7 with the pictures illustrating "fat" and "sun."
9. Place the child's letter squares at the top of the work space and give the child the Activity Page with the pictures illustrating "map," "fan," and "sit." Say, "Now you pick the letters for the first and last sounds in the words for these pictures."
10. Continue: "The word for this picture is 'map.' What is this?" After the child repeats "map," say, "Pick the letter for the beginning sound and tape [glue] it here (*point to the first line to the right of the map*)."
11. Continue: "Now say 'map' again, and pick the letter for the ending sound and tape [glue] it here (*point to the third line to the right of the picture*)." You may need to model saying the word slowly in order to help the child identify the final sound.
12. Teacher: "Let's check the sounds and letters: /m/ (*point to the m*), /a/ (*point to the middle line*), /p/ (*point to the p*)—'map.' Now you point to the letters as you say the word just as I did."
13. Repeat the procedure in steps 10, 11, and 12 with the pictures illustrating "fan" and "sit."
14. At the completion of the lesson, allow the child to choose a sticker and check the Progress Chart for Lesson 14.

Note: The Activity Page may need to be presented in another lesson if the child requires a lot of guidance and corrective feedback on the first part.

Teacher's Pictures and Letters: Beginning Letters *m*, *s*, *f* and Ending Letters *n*, *p*, *t* (Lesson 14)

m	s	f
n	p	t

Child's Letters: Letters *m*, *s*, and *f* for Beginning Sounds (Lesson 14)

m	s	f
n	p	t

Activity Page (Lesson 14)

Name _____

Beginning and Ending Letters

_____ _____ _____

_____ _____ _____

_____ _____ _____

Lesson 15: Beginning Letters *n*, *p*, *t* and Ending Letters *n*, *p*, *t*

Preparation

1. Copy and cut the teacher's page for Lesson 15.
2. Copy and cut the child's letter squares page and the Activity Page (Lesson 15) for each child.

Procedure

1. Place the teacher's letter and blank squares at the top of the work space.
2. Lay out in a column beneath the letters the pictures of a nap, a fin, and the number ten.
3. Teacher: "Today we are going to use these letters for the first and last sound in each of the words for these pictures. Let's begin with 'nap.'"
4. Continue: "The first sound in 'nap' is /n/, so I'll put *n* here (*to the right of the picture for 'nap'*). Next I'll put this (*a blank square*) for the /a/, and then *p* for the /p/." Say "nap" slowly, and point to each square as you say the sound.
5. Repeat the procedure in step 4 with the pictures of the fin and the number ten.
6. Remove the letter and blank squares and replace at the top of the work space. Say, "Now you do the first and last sounds for each of the words just as I did."
7. Pointing to the picture of the nap, say, "Tell me the word for this picture. . . . Now tell me just the first sound." After the child says /n/, say, "Now pick the letter for /n/ and place it here (*point to the right of the picture*). I'll put this (*a blank square*) for the /a/, and you pick the letter for /p/ and put it here (*point to the right of the blank square*)." Then say, "Let's check: /n/ (*point to the n*), /a/ (*point to the blank*), /p/ (*point to the p*)—nap."
8. Repeat the procedure in step 7 with the pictures of the fin and the number ten.
9. Place the child's letter squares at the top of the work space, and give the child the Activity Page with the pictures of the nut, the pan, and the top. Say, "Now you pick the letters for the first and last sounds in the words for these pictures."
10. Say, "The word for this picture is 'nut.' What is this?" After the child repeats 'nut,' say, "Pick the letter for the first sound, and tape [glue] it here (*point to the first line to the right of the nut*)."
11. Continue: "Now say 'nut' again, pick the letter for the ending sound, and tape [glue] it here (*point to the third line to the right of the picture*)." You may need to model saying the word slowly in order to help the child identify the final sound.
12. Say, "Let's check the sounds and letters: /n/ (*point to the n*) /u/ (*point to the middle line*), /t/ (*point to the t*)—nut. Now you point to the letters as you say the word just as I did."
13. Repeat the procedure in steps 10, 11, and 12 with the pictures of the top and the pan.
14. At the completion of the lesson, allow the child to choose a sticker and check the Progress Chart for Lesson 15.

Note: The Activity Page may need to be presented at the next lesson if progress is slow.

Teacher's Pictures and Letters: Beginning Letters *n*, *p*, *t* and Ending Letters *n*, *p*, *t* (Lesson 15)

n	p	t
n	p	n
		10

Child's Letters: Beginning Letters *n*, *p*, *t* and Ending Letters *n*, *p*, *t* (Lesson 15)

n	p	t
n	p	t

Activity Page (Lesson 15)

Name _____

Beginning and Ending Letters

_____   _____   _____

_____   _____   _____

_____   _____   _____

Lesson 16: Letters for Beginning and Ending Sounds

Preparation

1. Copy and cut the letters from teacher's page for Lesson 16; the bottom half of the sheet is used during the lesson.
2. Copy the Activity Page (Lesson 16) for each child.

Procedure

1. Place the letter squares for this lesson at the top of the work space.
2. Teacher: "Today you are going to pick the letters for the beginning and ending sounds in words without pictures. Let's try one."
3. Continue: "Our first word is 'mat': /m/, /a/, /t/. Pick the letter for /m/ and put it here (*point to the first line on the bottom half of the teacher's page*). Now listen for the ending sound: 'mat.' Pick the letter for the ending sound /t/ and put it here (*point to the third line*)."
4. Replace the letters at the top of the work space after the beginning and ending sounds are correctly selected for each word.
5. "Now you try one: 'fat.' Put the letter for the beginning sound here and the letter for the ending or last sound here (*point to the first and third lines*)." If the child has difficulty, say the word slowly and ask the child to pick the letter for the beginning sound. Then say it again and ask the child to pick the letter for the ending sound.
6. Words for identifying beginning and ending sounds:

mat, fat, pat	pit, pin, fun
sip, nip, tip	tip, tin, fat
tan, fan, man	sun, sit, sip
mat, man, map	

7. Continue with words for as long as the child is interested (as long as words with varying ending sounds have been included).
8. Give the child the Activity Page (Lesson 16).
9. Proceed: "Here are some words with the letters and sounds that we have been practicing. I think that you can read them. Let's see. The middle sound for each of these words is /a/. I'll show you how do it: /m/, /a/, /n/ (*point to each letter in sequence*)—man. Now you try this one (*point to the word 'pan'*)." Model (as above) if the child has difficulty. Continue through all of the words on the page or as long as the child is interested.
10. At the completion of the lesson, remind the child how much he or she has learned about the letters and sounds in words and that he or she can read some words with these letters and sounds. Tell the child to read the words on the page to someone at home—if indeed it is likely that he or she can do so independently. Allow the child to choose a sticker and check the Progress Chart for Lesson 16.

Note: The Activity Page may require a separate lesson, depending on the interest of the child and the amount of time used in the first part.

Teacher's Letters: Letters for Beginning and Ending Sounds (Lesson 16)

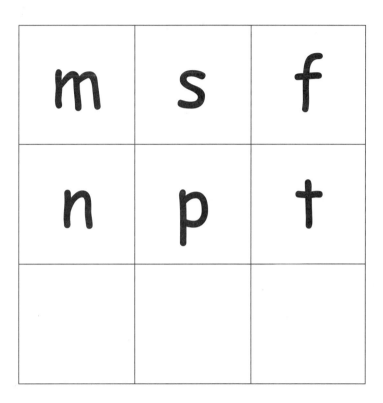

Lines for Beginning and Ending Sounds

Activity Page (Lesson 15)

Name _____

man	map	mat
fan	nap	fat
pan	tap	sat

man	fan	pan
mat	fat	pat
map		

tap

tan

sat

sap

Posttest and Take-Home Tiny Books

Preparation

1. Copy the assessment in Chapter 4 as a posttest for each child.
2. Copy and cut the tiny book pages for each child. Staple the left edge of each four-page book.

Procedure

1. Give posttest to each child following directions on the assessment.
2. When finished with the assessment say, "Now that we have finished our lessons, I have two tiny books which use the sounds and letters from our lessons. I'll help you read them at first. Then you can read them and take them home."
3. Model reading the first book by slowly saying the sound of each letter in the word while you smoothly track each letter with your finger. If the child joins in that is fine. (You may want to comment that the names in the book are silly but easy to sound out.)
4. Repeat step 3 but blend the sounds for each word more quickly.
5. Ask the child to read the book just as you did. Give the letter's sound immediately if the child hesitates.
6. Have child read it again.
7. Repeat steps 3–6 for the second book if the child is interested.
8. Teacher: "Now you may take these tiny books home to help you practice and remember the letters and sounds you have learned."
9. Score the child's posttest and enter the score on the Progress Chart.

Note: If the child's posttest score is below 24, the child is likely to need continued support in beginning reading instruction.

Child's Take-Home Tiny Book 1

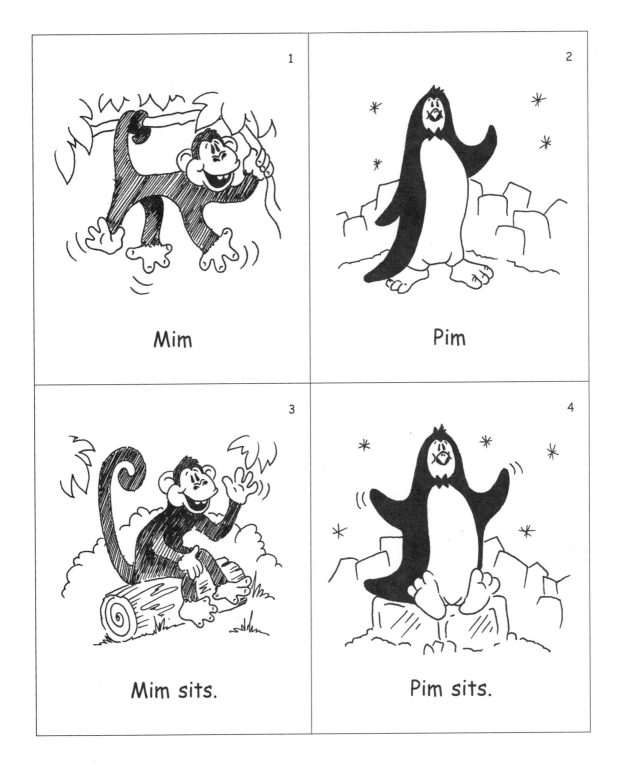

Child's Take-Home Tiny Book 2

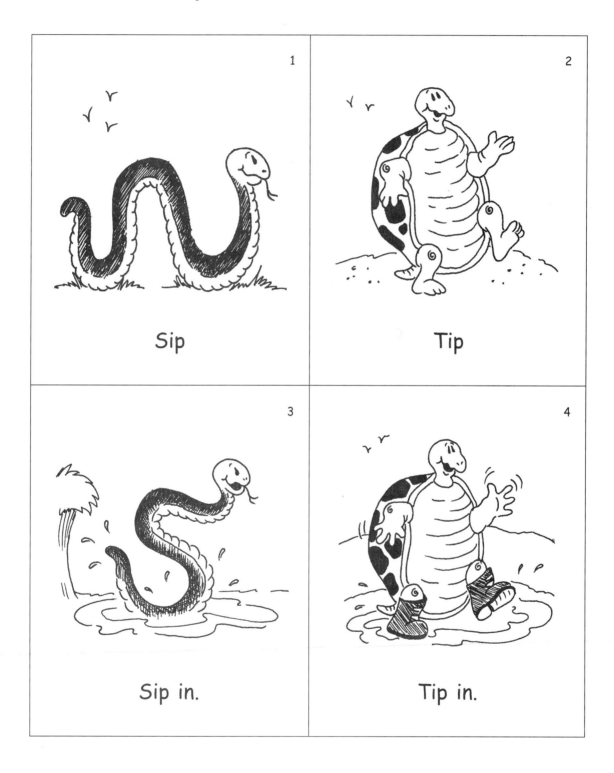

Chapter 6

Phoneme Characteristics and Lessons

Research clearly demonstrates that children who are taught language structure explicitly progress more readily in reading than those who are not (Moats & Lyon, 1996). Teachers should have knowledge of the characteristics of the phonemes (sounds) in English to assist children in comparing, contrasting, and differentiating them. Explicitly teaching phonemic awareness skills requires a fundamental understanding of phonemes. A phoneme is a basic sound segment in the lang ;e. For example, there are four phonemes (or sounds) in the word "frog": /f/, /r/, /o/, /g/.

IMPORTANCE OF UNDERSTANDING PHONEME PRODUCTION

Phonemic awareness instruction assists children in attending to the auditory characteristics of phonemes. Explicit discussion of how particular phonemes are made by the mouth enables children to understand better the similarities and differences between the phonemes. Individual phonemes are not perceptually salient acoustically, and sounds within words are strongly influenced by surrounding phonemes (coarticulation). The additional teaching of the motoric and visual cues of phonemes may be helpful in phoneme perception and identification. Many of you have probably observed children moving their mouths when trying to sound out a word or figure out the sounds to spell it. Researchers have stated that by helping children discover the articulatory positions, movements, and feel associated with phonemes, children experience a deeper level of phonological processing than by training that involves auditory awareness only (Howard, 1988; Lindamood & Lindamood, 1975, 1998; Skjelfjord, 1976). Becoming familiar with the place and manner of articulation assists children in anchoring the phonemes' identities (Damon, 1998).

PHONEMES IN WORDS

Phonemes can be complex and vary depending on the word. For example, in the word "crack," the lips are pursed or slightly rounded during the production of the initial sound "k." This is because the sound /r/ follows the /k/ and our lips are rounded for the production of /r./ In contrast, our lips are not slightly rounded for the production of initial /k/ in the word "kick." Neither sound that follows the /k/ require the lips to be protruded. The influence of sounds on other sounds in a word is called coarticulation. Additionally, some cautions about words containing two consonants in a row need to be discussed. Sometimes two letter spellings have one sound including the digraphs *ch, th, sh,* and numerous English orthographic spellings such as *ck, dg,* or *ph.* When two consonant sequences have two sounds, coarticulation (the influence of surrounding sounds) often changes the production and sound of the phoneme. For example, the /t/ in "truck" is produced differently and is much harder to perceive than the /t/ in a word beginning with a single consonant such as "top." At times the spelling of words do not reflect how each of the phonemes are produced in the word. For example, in the word "nose," the *se* is actually a /z/ sound. If the /s/ were produced in a blending task, children would be confused because /n/, /o/, /s/ does not form a word. Other common spelling/sound errors include past tense and plural spellings. For example, in the word "walked," the *ed* is actually a /t/ sound. In the word "dogs," the *s* is actually a /z/ sound; but in the word "cats," /s/ is the final sound.

SIMILARITIES BETWEEN PHONEMES

Children's errors when speaking, reading, and writing are often related to their difficulty discriminating among similar phonemes. Children may write "tite" for "kite" and be close to correct in regards to the characteristics of the sounds. The phonemes /t/ and /k/ are both produced with the voice turned off and by stopping the airflow briefly in the mouth before production of the sound. The only difference is in the location where the sound is made in the mouth (the place of articulation). The /t/ is produced with the tongue tip behind the front teeth, and the /k/ is produced by the back of the tongue in the back of our mouth. Children may also spell the word "pot" as "bot" because /p/ and /b/ are made exactly the same way by our mouths; we just turn our voice on a fraction of a second later when we say the /p/ sound in "pot" than when we say the /b/ sound in "bottle."

DESCRIPTION OF PHONEME PRODUCTION

Because of the complexity of phonemes, information about the classification of consonants may assist teachers in understanding the properties of phonemes (see Table 6.1). The consonant sounds have been described in detail to help teachers explain these complex properties of sounds to children during class lessons. Including explicit explanations about the acoustic features and production of the phonemes in the mouth together with traditional teaching regarding letter-sound associations when teaching the alphabet are very helpful in increasing children's awareness of phonemes.

Table 6.1 shows the 24 consonant sounds in the English language. There are 21 consonant letters in our alphabet. Three consonant letters do not have a distinctive sound (*c, x, q*). The *c* typically has a /k/ or /s/ sound, the *x* has the /k/ + /s/ sounds, and *q* has the /k/ or /k/ + /w/ sounds. Therefore, there are 18 consonant letters that represent distinctive sounds and 24 consonant sounds in the English language. The additional consonant sounds are /θ/ (voiceless *th*), /ð/ (voiced *th*), /ʃ/ (*sh*), /ʒ/ (*zh*), /tʃ/ (*ch*), /ŋ/ (*ng*).

Table 6.1 presents the 24 consonant sounds in English, indicating the place, manner, and voicing characteristics of each phoneme: the *place of articulation* tells us where in the mouth a sound is produced; the *manner of articulation* tells us how a sound is produced; and *voicing* tells us whether the sound requires the vocal folds to vibrate or not. For example, the sound /p/, as in "pie" and "ape," is described as a voiceless, bilabial, stop consonant. This description tells us that the sound is produced with the vocal folds not vibrating, the lips coming together (*bi* meaning "two" and *labia* meaning "lips"), and with a complete closure (stopping) of the airflow behind the lips before production of the sound.

English consonant sounds can be described by the following classification:

Voice	*Place*	*Manner*
Voiced	Bilabial	Stop
Voiceless	Labiodental	Nasal
	Interdental	Fricative
	Alveolar	Affricate
	Palatal	Liquid
	Velar	Glide
	Glottal	

Voicing of Phoneme Production

Each consonant sound in our language is produced with or without voicing. Fifteen sounds are produced with voicing, and nine are produced without voicing. Children often understand this concept by being told that our voice "motors" are on (voiced) or off (voiceless). By having children place a

TABLE 6.1. Consonant Classification by Place, Manner, and Voicing

Manner	Place						
	Bilabial (two lips)	Labiodental (top lip and teeth)	Linguadental (tongue and teeth)	Alveolar (ridge behind teeth)	Palatal (middle of mouth)	Velar (back of mouth)	Glottal (throat)
	Voicing − +	Voicing − +	Voicing − +	Voicing − +	Voicing − +	Voicing − +	Voicing − +
Stop (air stops)	/p/ /b/			/t/ /d/		/k/ /g/ (go)	
Fricative (continuous noisy air blowing)		/f/ /v/	/θ/ /ð/ (th) (th) thumb the	/s/ /z/	/ʃ/ /ʒ/ (sh) (zh) measure		/h/
Affricate (stop + noisy air)					/tʃ/ /dʒ/ (ch) (j) judge		
Nasal (sound through nose)	/m/			/n/		/ŋ/ (ng) ring	
Glide (quick sound)	/w/				/j/ (y) yellow		
Liquids				/l/	/r/		

hand on the throat area, they can feel whether the voice is on or off. For example, when /s/ and /z/ are compared, the only difference is that the motor is off for /s/ and on for /z/. Nine consonant sounds are produced without voicing and basically sound like a whisper. These sounds include /p/, /f/, /t/, /ʃ/ (*sh*), /s/, /k/, /θ/ (voiceless *th*), /tʃ/ (*ch*), and /h/. When we teach children about the voiceless sounds, it is helpful to blow a little more air out than usual for them to hear the sounds. One of the most common errors when we are pronouncing quiet sounds is to add a vowel (usually the sound /uh/, schwa vowel) after the sound. Adding the vowel makes the sound seem louder so that children will hear it. For example, the sound that the letter *s* makes is a long, continuous stream of air: /sssss/. Because it is a quiet, voiceless sound, some people mistakenly say the sound the letter *s* makes as /sssss uh/. Remember to forcefully blow the air out for emphasis on these sounds; do not turn the voice on or add the schwa vowel.

Most consonant sounds are produced with voicing. These sounds include /b/, /v/, /d/, /z/, /g/, /r/, /l/, /j/, /w/, /m/, /n/, /ð/ (voiced *th*) and /ŋ/ (*ng*). Special attention is needed when the voiced sounds are produced because it is impossible to produce some voiced sounds without a bit of a schwa vowel following them when they are produced in isolation. For example, if we incorrectly teach children that the production of the phoneme /d/ is /duh/ instead of saying the sound /d/ without lengthening the vowel after it, children will be confused when they start to blend sounds into words. Blending /duh/, /i/, /g/ sounds like a two-syllable word "/duh/-ig," not "dig."

Many of the sounds in our language only differ by voicing. Table 6.1 shows eight pairs of phonemes that only differ by voicing (/p/–/b/, /t/–/d/, /k/–/g/, /f/–/v/, /s/–/z/, /tʃ/–/dʒ/ (*ch–dg*), /θ/–/ð/ (voiceless and voiced *th*), /ʃ/–/ʒ/ (*sh–zh*).

Place of Phoneme Production

There are seven different places of articulation. These places of articulation proceed from the front of the mouth to the back of the mouth (see Table 6.1). Discussing which parts of our mouth are used to say the different sounds help children explore the properties of sounds. For example, the hard /g/ sound (as in "ga") is produced in the back of our mouth with the back of the tongue and the roof of the mouth. In contrast, the /b/ sound is produced in the front of the mouth with both lips.

Manner of Phoneme Production

There are six different manners of articulation. The description of the manner in which we say different sounds can also assist children in differentiating among phonemes. Some sounds are short, quick, quiet; others are long, hissy, loud, etc. For example, the /s/ sound is a long, hissy sound in which we blow the air through a small opening with our tongue. In contrast, the /t/ sound is a short, quick sound in which the air is stopped briefly and then forced out as the tongue is released.

The sounds in the English language that can be drawn out include /m/, /n/, /f/, /v/, /ʃ/ (*sh*), /s/, /z/, /θ/ (voiceless *th*), /ð/ (voiced *th*), /l/, /r/, and /h/. These phonemes can all be prolonged without affecting the production.

Many of the consonants in our language are brief because we stop the air and quickly blow it out to make these sounds. They include /p/, /b/, /t/, /d/, /k/, /g/, /tʃ/ (*ch*), and /dʒ/ (*dg*). These sounds cannot be drawn out, so be careful not to add the schwa vowel in an attempt to lengthen it. If you need to emphasize the sound, it is better to repeat the sound in isolation and then add the word. For example, /p/, /p/, /p/ "pie" would be better than adding the schwa vowel to the consonant, "/puh/-ie."

Additional information for the teacher as well as instruction and exercises for the class about the consonant phonemes are given below. These explicit explanations and lessons about the acoustic features and production of the phonemes should supplement alphabetic letter-sound instruction. For example, before or during instruction of the letter *d*, present the lesson for the phoneme /d/ to the whole class. Information about the articulatory and acoustic characteristics of the /d/ phoneme can then be discussed as opportunities arise (e.g., when a child makes an error in hearing the sound in a word or when you are presenting a book with frequent occurrences of the /d/ sound). Also, consider discussing questions or concerns about the properties of phonemes with a speech–language pathologist or other professional who may have studied linguistics, phonetics, and/or phonology.

LESSONS FOR SPECIFIC PHONEMES

The following lessons for each phoneme begin with information regarding articulatory features and common spellings of the phoneme for the teacher. Next, scripted information is included to describe the articulatory production to the class. An exercise in which children identify the target phoneme in isolation by listening and looking for the phoneme follows. Then children are required to discriminate which words begin with the target phoneme. Finally children are asked to identify whether the target phoneme occurs in the beginning, middle, or end of words. This task may be difficult for some children, and you can judge whether it is best to present this part of the lesson to the whole class or in small groups. The phoneme /ʒ/ is not included with these lessons because the sound occurs infrequently in our language.

REFERENCES

Damon, W. (Ed.). (1998). *Handbook of child psychology*. New York: Wiley.

Howard, M. (1998). Phonology first: A natural approach to beginning reading. *Idaho Reading Report, 31*, 123–134.

Lindamood, C. H., & Lindamood, P. C. (1975). *The A.D.D. program, auditory discrimination in depth*. Hingham, MA: Teaching Resources Corporation.

Lindamood, C. H., & Lindamood, P. C. (1998). *The Lindamood phoneme sequencing program for reading, spelling, and speech* (3rd ed.). Austin, TX: PRO-ED.

Moats, L. C., & Lyon, G. R. (1996). Wanted: Teachers with knowledge of language. *Topics in Language Disorders, 16*(2), 73–86.

Skjelfjord, V. J. (1976). Teaching children to segment spoken words as an aid in learning to read. *Journal of Learning Disabilities, 9*, 297–'305.

Phoneme /b/ (Letter *b*)

Information for the Teacher

- Place: both lips (bilabial)
- Voicing: voice on (voiced)
- Manner: stop (air blocked then blown out)
- Common spellings: *b*-ball, *bb*-rubber, *pb*-cupboard

Information for the Children

- "Today we are talking about the /b/ sound. There is one letter that often makes the /b/ sound, the letter *b*."
- "I make the /b/ by putting my lips together. When my lips come apart quickly, the air blows out and I can hear my voice when I say it."
- "I say the /b/ sound when I say 'boo.'"
- "Listen and watch my mouth as I make the /b/ sound, /b/, /b/, /b/, /b/, /b/, /b/." (Spread your lips apart and then slowly close them when making the /b/ sound to exaggerate the movement.)
- "Now you practice saying the /b/ sound several times. Feel your lips touch together and come apart as you say it. I'll hand out some mirrors to pass around. Look in the mirror as you say /b/ two times, then pass the mirror to the next child."

Listening and Looking for the /b/ Sound by Itself

- "Nod your head yes if you hear the /b/ sound. Shake your head no if you don't hear the /b/ sound."
- "/b/ (*pause*) Yes, that was the /b/ sound."
- "/s/ (*pause*) No, that was not the /b/ sound."
- "/m/ (*pause*) No, that was not the /b/ sound."
- "/b/ (*pause*) Yes, that was the /b/ sound."
- "/k/ (*pause*) No, that was not the /b/ sound."
- "/p/ (*pause*) That is a hard one. It's not the /b/ sound. We make the /p/ sound just like the /b/ sound, but the /p/ sound is a quiet sound. We have our voice off when we say the /p/ sound, but the /b/ is a loud sound with our voice on. Listen again to the difference between /b/ and /p/: /p/ is quiet; /b/ is louder with our voice on."
- "/f/ (*pause*) No, that was not the /b/ sound."
- "/b/ (*pause*) Yes, that was the /b/ sound."
- "/d/ (*pause*) No, that was not the /b/ sound." (If any children have nodded their heads indicating that it was the /b/ sound, explain that /d/ is a loud sound that blows air out like the /b/ sound but the /d/ sound is different because the front tip of the tongue goes up behind the front teeth instead of the lips coming together. Compare /d/ and /b/ again with special atten-

tion to how the mouth and lips move. Open your mouth a little more for the /d/ to let the children see where the tongue is placed for the /d/ sound. Ask the children to repeat /d/ and /b/ and to feel how their tongues and lips move differently for the two sounds.)

Listening and Looking for /b/ in the Beginning of Words

- "Now we're going to listen for the /b/ sound in words. Nod your head yes if /b/ is the first sound in the word I say. Shake your head no if you don't hear /b/ at the beginning of the word."
- "bat (*pause*) Yes, I hear the sound /b/ at the beginning of 'bat.' "
- "ball (*pause*) Yes, I hear the sound /b/ at the beginning of 'ball.' "
- "mop (*pause*) No, I don't hear the sound /b/ at the beginning of 'mop.' " (Emphasize /m/ a little extra.)
- "busy (*pause*) Yes, I hear /b/ at the beginning of 'busy.' "
- "some (*pause*) No, I don't hear /b/ at the beginning of 'some.' "
- "tall (*pause*) No, I don't hear /b/ at the beginning of 'tall.' "
- "borrow (*pause*) Yes, I hear /b/ at the beginning of 'borrow.' "

Listening and Looking for /b/ in the Beginning, Middle, or End of Words

- "Now all the words I say are going to have the sound /b/ in the word, but you have to listen very carefully and watch my mouth as I say the words. When I call on you, your job will be to tell me if you heard the sound /b/ in the beginning (first sound), middle, or end (last sound) of the word. For example, if I say the word 'cube,' the /b/ sound is at the end of the word. 'Cube'—hear the /b/ at the end? If I say 'bug,' the /b/ sound is the beginning sound in the word."
- cab (end)
- job (end)
- boat (beginning)
- globe (end)
- burn (beginning)
- above (middle)
- bus (beginning)
- knob (end)
- rib (end)
- boot (beginning)
- hobby (middle)
- beard (beginning)

Phoneme /k/ (Letters *c, k*)

Information for the Teacher

- Place: back of mouth (velar)
- Voicing: quiet (voiceless)
- Manner: stop (air blocked, then blown out)
- Common spellings: *k*-kite, *c*-cat, *ck*-back, x(*ks*)-box, q(*kw*)-quiet

Information for the Children

- "Today we are talking about the /k/ sound. There are two different letters that often make the /k/ sound: the letter *c* and the letter *k*."
- "I make the /k/ with the back of my tongue touching the back of the roof of my mouth. When my tongue drops down a little, the air blows out: /k/ is a quiet sound. I just hear air blowing, I don't hear my voice on when I say it."
- "Listen and watch my mouth as I make the /k/ sound: /k/, /k/, /k/, /k/, /k/, /k/, /k/." (Open your mouth a little wider than usual for a couple of /k/ productions so that children can see the back of your tongue moving up and down as you say the sound.)
- "Now you practice saying the /k/ sound several times. Feel where your tongue goes in your mouth as you say it. I'll hand out some mirrors to pass around. Look in the mirror as you say /k/ two times, then pass the mirror to the next child."

Listening and Looking for the /k/ Sound by Itself

- "Nod your head yes if you hear the /k/ sound. Shake your head no if you don't hear the /k/ sound."
- "/k/ (*pause*) Yes, that was the /k/ sound."
- "/s/ (*pause*) No, that was not the /k/ sound."
- "/m/ (*pause*) No that was not the /k/ sound."
- "/k/ (*pause*) Yes, that was the /k/ sound."
- "/g/ (*pause*) That is a hard one. It's not the /k/ sound. We make the /g/ sound somewhat like the /k/ sound, but the /g/ sound is a loud sound. We have our voice on when we say the /g/ sound, but the /k/ is a quiet sound with our voice off. Listen again to the difference between /k/ and /g/: /k/ is quiet; /g/ is louder with our voice on."
- "/f/ (*pause*) No, that was not the /k/ sound."
- "/k/ (*pause*) Yes, that was the /k/ sound."
- "/t/ (*pause*) No, that was not the /k/ sound." (If any children have nodded their heads indicating that it was the /k/ sound, explain that /t/ is a quiet sound that blows air out like the /k/ sound but the /t/ sound is different because the front tip of the tongue goes up behind the front teeth instead of the back of the tongue going up for /k/. Compare /t/ and /k/ again with your mouth slightly more open than usual so that the children can see the difference in which

part of your tongue moves as you say those sounds. Ask the children to repeat /t/ and /k/ and to feel how their tongue moves differently for the two sounds.)

Listening and Looking for /k/ in the Beginning of Words

- "Now we're going to listen for the /k/ sound in words. Nod your head yes if /k/ is the first sound in the word I say. Shake your head no if you don't hear /k/ at the beginning of the word."
- "car (*pause*) Yes, I hear the sound /k/ at the beginning of 'car.'"
- "kite (*pause*) Yes, I hear the sound /k/ at the beginning of 'kite.'"
- "mop (*pause*) No, I don't hear the sound /k/ at the beginning of 'mop.'"
- "castle (*pause*) Yes, I hear /k/ at the beginning of 'castle.'"
- "fun (*pause*) No, I don't hear /k/ at the beginning of 'fun.'"
- "toe (*pause*) No, I don't hear /k/ at the beginning of 'toe.'"
- "cold (*pause*) Yes, I hear /k/ at the beginning of 'cold.'"

Listening and Looking for /k/ in the Beginning, Middle, or End of Words

- "Now all the words I say are going to have the sound /k/ in the word, but you have to listen very carefully and watch my mouth as I say the words. When I call on someone, your job will be to tell me if you heard the sound /k/ at the beginning (first sound), middle, or end (last sound) of the word. For example, if I say the word 'block,' the /k/ sound is at the end of the word. 'Block'—hear the /k/ at the end? If I say 'king,' the /k/ sound is the beginning sound in the word."
- Luke (end)
- sack (end)
- cap (beginning)
- trick (end)
- Kyle (beginning)
- bucket (middle)
- camera (beginning)
- luck (end)
- rake (end)
- kid (beginning)
- racket (middle)
- coffee (beginning)

Phoneme /d/ (Letter *d*)

Information for the Teacher

- Place: tongue on ridge behind front top teeth (alveolar ridge)
- Voicing: voice on (voiced)
- Manner: stop (air blocked, then blown out)
- Common spellings: *d*-door, *dd*-ladder, *ed*-called, *ld*-could

Information for the Children

- "Today we are talking about the /d/ sound. There is one letter that often makes the /d/ sound, the letter *d*."
- "I make the /d/ with the front of my tongue touching the bumpy place behind my top front teeth. When my tongue tip drops down a little, the air blows out. The /d/ sound is a loud sound because I hear my voice on when I say it."
- "Listen and watch my mouth as I make the /d/ sound: /d/, /d/, /d/, /d/, /d/, /d/, /d/." (Open your mouth a little wider than usual for a couple of /d/ productions so that children can see the front of your tongue moving up and down as you say the sound.)
- "Now you practice saying the /d/ sound several times. Feel where your tongue goes in your mouth as you say it. I'll hand out some mirrors to pass around. Look in the mirror as you say /d/ two times, then pass the mirror to the next child."

Listening and Looking for the /d/ Sound by Itself

- "Nod your head yes if you hear the /d/ sound. Shake your head no if you don't hear the /d/ sound."
- "/d/ (*pause*) Yes, that was the /d/ sound."
- "/s/ (*pause*) No, that was not the /d/ sound."
- "/n/ (*pause*) No, that was not the /d/ sound."
- "/d/ (*pause*) Yes, that was the /d/ sound."
- "/t/ (*pause*) That is a hard one. It's not the /d/ sound. We make the /d/ sound somewhat like the /t/ sound, but the /d/ sound is a loud sound. We have our voice on when we say the /d/ sound, but the /t/ is a quiet sound with our voice off. Listen again to the difference between /t/ and /d/: /t/ is quiet; /d/ is louder with our voice on."
- "/f/ (*pause*) No, that was not the /d/ sound."
- "/d/ (*pause*) Yes, that was the /d/ sound."
- "/g/ (*pause*) No, that was not the /d/ sound." (If any children have nodded their heads indicating that it was the /d/ sound, explain that /g/ is a loud sound that blows air out like the /d/ sound but the /g/ sound is different because the back of tongue goes up for /g/ and the front tip of the tongue goes up behind the front teeth for /d/. Compare /d/ and /g/ again with your mouth slightly more open than usual so that the children can see the different ways in which

part of your tongue moves as you say those sounds. Ask the children to repeat /d/ and /g/ and to feel how their tongues move differently for the two sounds.)

Listening and Looking for /d/ in the Beginning of Words

- "Now we're going to listen for the /d/ sound in words. Nod your head yes if /d/ is the first sound in the word I say. Shake your head no if you don't hear /d/ at the beginning of the word."
- "doll (*pause*) Yes, I hear the sound /d/ at the beginning of 'doll.' "
- "door (*pause*) Yes, I hear the sound /d/ at the beginning of 'door.' "
- "nose (*pause*) No, I don't hear the sound /d/ at the beginning of 'nose.' " (Emphasize /n/ a little extra.)
- "doghouse (*pause*) Yes, I hear /d/ at the beginning of 'doghouse.' "
- "bubble (*pause*) No, I don't hear /d/ at the beginning of 'bubble.' "
- "finger (*pause*) No, I don't hear /d/ at the beginning of 'finger.' "
- "daylight (*pause*) Yes, I hear /d/ at the beginning of 'daylight.' "

Listening and Looking for /d/ in the Beginning, Middle, or End of Words

- "Now all the words I say are going to have the sound /d/ in the word, but you have to listen very carefully and watch my mouth as I say the words. When I call on you, your job will be to tell me if you heard the sound /d/ at the beginning (first sound), middle, or end (last sound) of the word. For example, if I say the word 'bed,' the /d/ sound is at the end of the word. 'Bed'— hear the /d/ at the end? If I say 'dance,' the /d/ sound is the beginning sound in the word."
- bad (end)
- played (end)
- dog (beginning)
- odd (end)
- dairy (beginning)
- body (middle)
- doorstep (beginning)
- lid (end)
- lemonade (end)
- down (beginning)
- hidden (middle)
- dip (beginning)

Phoneme /f/ (Letter *f*)

Information for the Teacher

- Place: top teeth on bottom lip (labiodental)
- Voicing: quiet (voiceless)
- Manner: fricative (noisy air continuously blowing out)
- Common spellings: *f*-feet, *gh*-laugh, *ff*-waffle, *ph*-phone

Information for the Children

- "Today we are talking about the /f/ sound. The letter *f* makes the /f/ sound."
- "I make the /f/ with my top teeth touching my bottom lip while I'm blowing air out. The /f/ sound is a quiet sound. I just hear air blowing—I don't hear my voice on when I say it."
- "Listen and watch my mouth as I make the /f/ sound: /f/, /f/, /f/, /f/, /f/, /f/, /f/." Drag the sound out as you say it.
- "Now you practice saying the /f/ sound several times. Feel where your top teeth touch your bottom lip as you say it. I'll hand out some mirrors to pass around. Look in the mirror as you say /f/ two times, then pass the mirror to the next child."

Listening and Looking for the /f/ Sound by Itself

- "Watch my mouth and listen carefully as I say some sounds. Nod your head yes if you hear and see the /f/ sound. Shake your head no if you don't hear the /f/ sound."
- "/f/ (*pause*) Yes, that was the /f/ sound."
- "/r/ (*pause*) No, that was not the /f/ sound."
- "/m/ (*pause*) No, that was not the /f/ sound."
- "/f/ (*pause*) Yes, that was the /f/ sound."
- "/v/ (*pause*) That is a hard one. It's not the /f/ sound. We make the /v/ sound somewhat like the /f/ sound, but the /v/ sound is a loud sound. We have our voice on when we say the /v/ sound, but /f/ is a quiet sound with our voice off. Listen again to the difference /f/ and /v/: /f/ is quiet; /v/ is louder with our voice on."
- "/k/ (*pause*) No, that was not the /f/ sound."
- "/f/ (*pause*) Yes, that was the /f/ sound."
- "/s/ (*pause*) No, that was not the /f/ sound." (If any children have nodded their heads indicating that it was the /f/ sound, explain that /s/ is a quiet sound that blows air out like the /f/ sound but the /s/ sound is different because the front tip of the tongue goes up behind the front teeth instead of the top teeth touching the bottom lip for /f/. Compare /s/ and /f/ again, pointing to your mouth as you say the sounds so that the children can see the difference in what moves as you say those sounds. Ask the children to repeat /s/ and /f/ and to feel how their mouths move differently for the two sounds.)

Listening and Looking for /f/ in the Beginning of Words

- "Now we're going to listen and look for the /f/ sound in words. Watch my mouth as I say these words. Nod your head yes if /f/ is the first sound in the word I say. Shake your head no if you don't hear /f/ at the beginning of the word."
- "foot (*pause*) Yes, I hear the sound /f/ at the beginning of foot."
- "fire (*pause*) Yes, I hear the sound /f/ at the beginning of fire."
- "shoe (*pause*) No, I don't hear the sound /f/ at the beginning of shoe." (Emphasize /ʃ/ a little extra.)
- "Friday (*pause*) Yes, I hear /f/ at the beginning of Friday."
- "jump (*pause*) No, I don't hear /f/ at the beginning of jump."
- "sister (*pause*) No, I don't hear /f/ at the beginning of sister."
- "fantastic (*pause*) Yes, I hear /f/ at the beginning of fantastic."

Listening and Looking for /f/ in the Beginning, Middle, or End of Words

- "Now all the words I say are going to have the sound /f/ in the word, but you have to listen very carefully and watch my mouth as I say the words. When I call on you, your job will be to tell me if you heard the sound /f/ at the beginning (first sound), middle, or end (last sound) of the word. For example, if I say the word 'rough,' the /f/ sound is at the end of the word. 'Rough'—hear the /f/ at the end? If I say 'finger,' the /f/ sound is the beginning sound in the word."
- awful (middle)
- laugh (end)
- first (beginning)
- often (middle)
- feeling (beginning)
- tough (end)
- off (end)
- coffee (middle)
- fun (beginning)
- muffin (middle)
- phone (beginning)
- wolf (end)

Phoneme /g/ (Letter g)

Information for the Teacher

- Place: back of mouth (velar)
- Voicing: voice on (voiced)
- Manner: stop (air blocked then blown out)
- Common spellings: g-goat, gg-egg

Information for the Children

- "Today we are talking about the /g/ sound. The letter g makes the /g/ sound."
- "I make the /g/ with the back of my tongue touching the back of the roof of my mouth. When my tongue drops down a little, I turn my voice on and the air blows out. The /g/ sound is a loud sound. I hear my voice on—I feel the voice if I put my hand on my throat when I say /g/."
- "Listen and watch my mouth as I make the /g/ sound: /g/, /g/, /g/, /g/, /g/, /g/, /g/." (Open your mouth a little wider than usual for a couple /g/ productions so that children can see the back of your tongue moving up and down as you say the sound.)
- "Now you practice saying the /g/ sound several times. Feel where your tongue goes in your mouth as you say it. Feel your neck and throat to feel your voice turned on as you say /g/. I'll hand out some mirrors to pass around. Look in the mirror as you say /g/ two times, then pass the mirror to the next child."

Listening and Looking for the /g/ Sound by Itself

- "Nod your head yes if you hear the /g/ sound. Shake your head no if you don't hear the /g/ sound."
- "/g/ (pause) Yes, that was the /g/ sound."
- "/v/ (pause) No, that was not the /g/ sound."
- "/n/ (pause) No, that was not the /g/ sound."
- "/g/ (pause) Yes, that was the /g/ sound."
- "/k/ (pause) That is a hard one. It's not the /g/ sound. We make the /g/ sound somewhat like the /k/ sound, but the /g/ sound is a loud sound. We have our voice on when we say the /g/ sound, but the /k/ is a quiet sound with our voice off. Listen again to the difference between /k/ and /g/: /k/ is quiet; /g/ is louder with our voice on."
- "/l/ (pause) No, that was not the /g/ sound."
- "/g/ (pause) Yes, that was the /g/ sound."
- "/d/ (pause) No, that was not the /g/ sound." (If any children nod their heads indicating that it was the /g/ sound, explain that /d/ is a loud sound that blows air out like the /g/ sound but the /d/ sound is different because the front tip of the tongue goes up behind the front teeth instead of the back of the tongue going up for /g/. Compare /d/ and /g/ again with your mouth

slightly more open than usual so that the children can see the difference in which part of your tongue moves as you say those sounds. Ask the children to repeat /d/ and /g/ and to feel how their tongues move differently for the two sounds.)

Listening and Looking for /g/ in the Beginning of Words

- "Now we're going to listen for the /g/ sound in words. Nod your head yes if /g/ is the first sound in the word I say. Shake your head no if you don't hear /g/ at the beginning of the word."
- "game (*pause*) Yes, I hear the sound /g/ at the beginning of 'game.'"
- "golf (*pause*) Yes, I hear the sound /g/ at the beginning of 'golf.'"
- "sun (*pause*) No, I don't hear the sound /g/ at the beginning of 'sun.'"
- "gone (*pause*) Yes, I hear /g/ at the beginning of 'gone.'"
- "fun (*pause*) No, I don't hear /g/ at the beginning of 'fun.'"
- "dance (*pause*) No, I don't hear /g/ at the beginning of 'dance.'"
- "ghost (*pause*) Yes, I hear /g/ at the beginning of 'ghost.'"

Listening and Looking for /g/ in the Beginning, Middle, or End of Words

- "Now all the words I say are going to have the sound /g/ in the word, but you have to listen very carefully and watch my mouth as I say the words. When I call on you, your job will be to tell me if you heard the sound /g/ at the beginning (first sound), middle, or end (last sound) of the word. For example, if I say the word 'rug,' the /g/ sound is at the end of the word. 'Rug'—hear the /g/ at the end? If I say 'goal,' the /g/ sound is the beginning sound in the word."
- gum (beginning)
- leg (end)
- frog (end)
- foggy (middle)
- tiger (middle)
- bug (end)
- gas (beginning)
- wagon (middle)
- go (beginning)
- wiggle (middle)
- gate (beginning)
- dog (end)

Phoneme /h/ (Letter *h*)

Information for the Teacher

- Place: in the throat (glottal)
- Voicing: quiet (voiceless)
- Manner: fricative (noisy air continuously blowing out)
- Common spellings: *h*-happy, *wh*-who

Information for the Children

- "Today we are talking about the /h/ sound. The letter *h* makes the /h/ sound."
- "I make the /h/ with the my lips open a little bit and my tongue down. Then I blow air through my throat right here (*point to middle of your neck*). The /h/ sound is a quiet sound. I just hear air blowing, I don't hear my voice on when I say it."
- "/h/ is the sound we make for things that are hot. If we eat something that is too hot, we might say /h/, /h/, /h/ot."
- "Listen and watch my mouth as I make the /h/ sound: /h/, /h/, /h/, /h/, /h/, /h/, /h/."
- "Now you practice saying the /h/ sound several times. Feel the air blow quietly through your mouth. Your mouth just has to open a little bit to make the /h/ sound. Your tongue or your lips don't really have to move. I'll hand out some mirrors to pass around. Look in the mirror as you say /h/ two times, then pass the mirror to the next child."

Listening and Looking for the /h/ Sound by Itself

- "Watch my mouth and listen carefully as I say some sounds. Nod your head yes if you hear the /h/ sound. Shake your head no if you don't hear the /h/ sound."
- "/h/ (*pause*) Yes, that was the /h/ sound."
- "/s/ (*pause*) No, that was not the /h/ sound."
- "/m/ (*pause*) No, that was not the /h/ sound."
- "/h/ (*pause*) Yes, that was the /h/ sound."
- "/w/ (*pause*) No, that was not the /h/ sound."
- "/k/ (*pause*) No, that was not the /s/ sound."
- "/h/ (*pause*) Yes, that was the /h/ sound."
- "/f/ (*pause*) No, that was not the /h/ sound." (If any children have nodded their heads indicating that it was the /h/ sound, explain that /f/ is a quiet sound that blows air out like the /h/ sound but the /f/ sound is different because the top teeth touch the bottom lip whereas the /h/ sound is made in the throat. Compare /h/ and /f/ again, with you pointing to your mouth as you say the sounds so that the children can see the difference in what moves as you say those sounds. Ask the children to repeat /h/ and /f/ and to feel how their mouths move differently for the two sounds.)

Listening and Looking for /h/ in the Beginning of Words

- "Now we're going to listen and look for the /h/ sound in words. Watch my mouth as I say these words. Nod your head yes if /h/ is the first sound in the word I say. Shake your head no if you don't hear /h/ at the beginning of the word."
- "hide (*pause*) Yes, I hear the sound /h/ at the beginning of 'hide.'"
- "happy (*pause*) Yes, I hear the sound /h/ at the beginning of 'happy.'"
- "fever (*pause*) No, I don't hear the sound /h/ at the beginning of 'fever.'" (Emphasize /f/ a little extra.)
- "hike (*pause*) Yes, I hear /h/ at the beginning of 'hike.'"
- "swimming (*pause*) No, I don't hear /h/ at the beginning of 'swimming.'"
- "sheep (*pause*) No, I don't hear /h/ at the beginning of 'sheep.'"
- "help (*pause*) Yes, I hear /h/ at the beginning of 'help.'"

Listening and Looking for /h/ in the Beginning, Middle, or End of Words

- "Now all the words I say are going to have the sound /h/ in the word, but you have to listen very carefully and watch my mouth as I say the words. When I call on you, your job will be to tell me if you heard the sound /h/ at the beginning (first sound) or middle (between other sounds) of the word. For example, if I say the word 'playhouse,' the /h/ sound is in the middle of the word. 'Playhouse'—hear the /h/ in the middle? If I say 'heel,' the /h/ sound is the beginning sound in the word."
- anyhow (middle)
- hold (beginning)
- behave (middle)
- holiday (beginning)
- rehearse (middle)
- hurricane (beginning)
- grasshopper (middle)
- home (beginning)
- horse (beginning)
- beehive (middle)

Phoneme /ʤ/ (Letter *j*, Digraph *dg*, Letter *g*)

Information for the Teacher

- Place: tongue half way back in your mouth (palatal)
- Voicing: voice on (voiced)
- Manner: affricate (air briefly blocked then noisy air blowing out)
- Common spellings: *j*-jacket, *dg*-budget, *ge*-college, *dge*-edge, *d*-gradual, *g*-magic

Information for the Children

- "Today we are talking about the /ʤ/ sound. The letters *j* or soft *g* make the /ʤ/ sound. When the /ʤ/ sound is at the middle or the end of words, the letters *g* or *dg* usually make the /ʤ/ sound."
- "I make the sound /ʤ/ with my tongue in the middle of my mouth. I then turn my voice on, blocking the air for a short time, then air blows out. The /ʤ/ sound is a loud sound. I hear my voice on when I say it."
- "Listen and watch my mouth as I make the /ʤ/ sound: /ʤ/, /ʤ/, /ʤ/, /ʤ/, /ʤ/, /ʤ/, /ʤ/."
- "Now you practice saying the /ʤ/ sound several times. Feel where your tongue is in the middle of your mouth. Feel how you turn on your voice, block the air, then air blows out just for a little bit. I'll hand out some mirrors to pass around. Look in the mirror as you say /ʤ/ two times, then pass the mirror to the next child."

Listening and Looking for the /ʤ/ Sound by Itself

- "Watch my mouth and listen carefully as I say some sounds. Nod your head yes if you hear and see the /ʤ/ sound. Shake your head no if you don't hear the /ʤ/ sound."
- "/ʤ/ (*pause*) Yes, that was the /ʤ/ sound."
- "/z/ (*pause*) No, that was not the /ʤ/ sound."
- "/ʧ/ (*ch*) (*pause*) That is a hard one. It's not the /ʤ/ sound. We make the /ʧ/ sound just like the /ʤ/ sound, but the /ʤ/ sound is a loud sound. We have our voice on when we say the /ʤ/ sound, but /ʧ/ is a quiet sound with our voice off. Listen again to the difference between /ʧ/ and /ʤ/: /ʧ/ is quiet; the /ʤ/ sound is louder with our voice on."
- "/ʤ/ (*pause*) Yes, that was the /ʤ/ sound."
- "/ʤ/ (*pause*) Yes, that was the /ʤ/ sound."
- "/ʃ/ (*sh*) (*pause*) No, that was not the /ʤ/ sound."
- "/d/ (*pause*) No, that was not the /ʤ/ sound." (If any children have nodded their heads indicating that it was the /ʤ/ sound, explain that /d/ is a loud sound like /ʤ/ but the /d/ sound is different because the tongue is right behind the front teeth and /d/ is a little shorter sound. For /ʤ/ the tongue is more in the middle of our mouth and it's a little longer and noisier

sound. Compare /d/ and /dʒ/ again. Ask the children to repeat /d/ and /dʒ/ and to feel how their tongues move differently for the two sounds.)

- "/dʒ/ (*pause*) Yes, that was the /dʒ/ sound."

Listening and Looking for /dʒ/ in the Beginning of Words

- "Now we're going to listen and look for the /dʒ/ sound in words. Watch my mouth as I say these words. Nod your head yes if /dʒ/ is the first sound in the word I say. Shake your head no if you don't hear /dʒ/ at the beginning of the word."
- "jelly (*pause*) Yes, I hear the sound /dʒ/ at the beginning of 'jelly.'"
- "jump (*pause*) Yes, I hear the sound /dʒ/ at the beginning of 'jump.'"
- "zipper (*pause*) No, I don't hear the sound /dʒ/ at the beginning of 'zipper.'"
- "juice (*pause*) Yes, I hear /dʒ/ at the beginning of 'juice.'"
- "shoe (*pause*) No, I don't hear /dʒ/ at the beginning of 'shoe.'"
- "summer (*pause*) No, I don't hear /dʒ/ at the beginning of 'summer.'"
- "joke (*pause*) Yes, I hear /dʒ/ at the beginning of 'joke.'"

Listening and Looking for /dʒ/ in the Beginning, Middle, or End of Words

- "Now all of the words I say are going to have the sound /dʒ/ in the word, but you have to listen very carefully and watch my mouth as I say the words. When I call on you, your job will be to tell me if you heard the sound /dʒ/ at the beginning (first sound), middle, or end (last sound) of the word. For example, if I say the word 'bridge,' the /dʒ/ sound is at the end of the word. 'Bridge'—hear /dʒ/ at the end? If I say 'job,' the /dʒ/ sound is the beginning sound in the word."
- June (beginning)
- large (end)
- college (end)
- soldier (middle)
- fudge (end)
- jam (beginning)
- imagine (middle)
- just (beginning)
- July (beginning)
- huge (end)
- change (end)

Phoneme /l/ (Letter *l*)

Information for the Teacher

- Place: tongue on ridge behind front top teeth (alveolar ridge)
- Voicing: voice on (voiced)
- Manner: liquid/ lateral (sound goes out on each side of tongue when making this sound)
- Common spellings: *l*-look, *ll*-ball

Information for the Children

- "Today we are talking about the /l/ sound. The letter *l* makes the /l/ sound."
- "I make the /l/ by holding the tip of my tongue behind my top front teeth while I turn on my voice. The /l/ sound is a loud sound. I hear my voice on when I say /l/."
- "Listen and watch my mouth as I make the /l/ sound: /l/, /l/, /l/, /l/, /l/, /l/."
- "Now you practice saying the /l/ sound several times. Feel where your tongue is behind your front teeth. Feel how you turn on your voice and keep your tongue up behind your teeth. I'll hand out some mirrors to pass around. Look in the mirror as you say /l/ two times, then pass the mirror to the next child."

Listening and Looking for the /l/ Sound by Itself

- "Watch my mouth and listen carefully as I say some sounds. Nod your head yes if you hear and see the /l/ sound. Shake your head no if you don't hear the /l/ sound."
- "/l/ (*pause*) Yes, that was the /l/ sound."
- "/r/ (*pause*) No, that was not the /l/ sound."
- "/w/ (*pause*) No, that was not the /l/ sound." (If any children have noded their heads indicating that it was the /l/ sound, explain that /w/ is a loud sound like /l/ but the /w/ sound is different because we pucker up and move our lips to say /w/ whereas for /l/ we leave our lips still and just move our tongue to behind our teeth. Compare /w/ and /l/ again. Ask the children to repeat /w/ and /l/ and feel how their mouths move differently for the two sounds.)
- "/l/ (*pause*) Yes, that was the /l/ sound."
- "/g/ (*pause*) No, that was not the /l/ sound."
- "/l/ (*pause*) Yes, that was the /l/ sound."
- "/j/ (*y*) (*pause*) No, that was not the /l/ sound." (If any children have nodded their heads indicating that it was the /l/ sound, explain that /j/ is a loud sound like /l/ but the /j/ sound is different because the middle of the tongue moves up a little whereas for /l/ the tip of the tongue moves up and stays touching behind the front teeth. Compare /j/ and /l/ again. Ask the children to repeat /j/ and /l/ and feel how their mouths move differently for the two sounds.)
- "/m/ (*pause*) No, that was not the /l/ sound."
- "/l/ (*pause*) Yes, that was the /l/ sound."

Listening and Looking for /l/ in the Beginning of Words

- "Now we're going to listen and look for the /l/ sound in words. Watch my mouth as I say these words. Nod your head yes if /l/ is the first sound in the word I say. Shake your head no if you don't hear /l/ at the beginning of the word."
- "lips (*pause*) Yes, I hear the sound /l/ at the beginning of 'lips.'"
- "love (*pause*) Yes, I hear the sound /l/ at the beginning of 'love.'"
- "window (*pause*) No, I don't hear the sound /l/ at the beginning of 'window.'"
- "late (*pause*) Yes, I hear /l/ at the beginning of 'late.'"
- "run (*pause*) No, I don't hear /l/ at the beginning of 'run.'"
- "you (*pause*) No, I don't hear /l/ at the beginning of 'you.'"
- "lion (*pause*) Yes, I hear /l/ at the beginning of 'lion.'"

Listening and Looking for /l/ in the Beginning, Middle, or End of Words

- "Now all of the words I say are going to have the sound /l/ in the word, but you have to listen very carefully and watch my mouth as I say the words. When I call on someone, your job will be to tell me if you heard the sound /l/ at the beginning (first sound), middle, or end (last sound) of the word. For example, if I say the word 'hall,' the /l/ sound is at the end of the word. 'Hall'—hear /l/ at the end? If I say 'lick,' the /l/ sound is the beginning sound in the word."
- lake (beginning)
- large (beginning)
- small (end)
- yellow (middle)
- mail (end)
- leaf (beginning)
- falling (middle)
- late (beginning)
- like (beginning)
- cool (end)
- tall (end)

Phoneme /m/ (Letter *m*)

Information for the Teacher

- Place: both lips (bilabial)
- Voicing: voice on (voiced)
- Manner: air passes through the nose (nasal)
- Common spellings: *m*-mat, *mm*-comment, *lm*-calm, *mb*-comb, *mn*-hymn

Information for the Children

- "Today we are talking about the /m/ sound. There is one letter that most often makes the /m/ sound: the letter *m*."
- "I make the /m/ by putting my lips together. I keep lips together and let the air come out of my nose. I can hear my voice when I say it, too."
- "The /m/ sound is the sound we make when we eat something that tastes really good. We say 'mmmmm.'"
- "Listen and watch my mouth as I make the /m/ sound: /m/, /m/, /m/, /m/, /m/, /m/, /m/."
- "Now you practice saying the /m/ sound several times. Feel your lips stay together as you say it. I'll hand out some mirrors to pass around. Look in the mirror as you say /m/ two times, then pass the mirror to the next child."

Listening and Looking for the /m/ Sound by Itself

- "Nod your head yes if you see and hear the /m/ sound. Shake your head no if you don't hear the /m/ sound."
- "/m/ (*pause*) Yes, that was the /m/ sound."
- "/s/ (*pause*) No, that was not the /m/ sound."
- "/k/ (*pause*) No, that was not the /m/ sound."
- "/m/ (*pause*) Yes, that was the /m/ sound."
- "/g/ (*pause*) No, that was not the /m/ sound."
- "/b/ (*pause*) That is a hard one. It's not the /m/ sound. We make the /b/ sound with our lips in the same place as the /m/ sound, but the /b/ sound is a short sound and we blow air out of our mouths. The /m/ sound is a long sound, and air comes out of my nose. Listen again to the difference between /b/ and /m/: /b/ is short and /m/ is long."
- "/f/ (*pause*) No, that was not the /m/ sound."
- "/m/ (*pause*) Yes, that was the /m/ sound."
- "/n/ (*pause*) No, that was not the /m/ sound." (If any children have nodded their heads indicating that it was the /m/ sound, explain that /n/ is a loud sound that blows air out of the nose like the /m/ sound but the /n/ sound is different because the front tip of the tongue goes up behind the front teeth instead of the lips coming together. Compare /n/ and /m/ again, with special attention to how the mouth and lips move. Open your mouth a little more for the /n/ to let the

children see where the tongue is placed for the /n/ sound. Ask the children to repeat /m/ and /n/ and to feel how their tongues and lips move differently for the two sounds.)

Listening and Looking for /m/ in the Beginning of Words

- "Now we're going to look and listen for the /m/ sound in words. Nod your head yes if /m/ is the first sound in the word I say. Shake your head no if you don't hear /m/ at the beginning of the word."
- "move (*pause*) Yes, I hear the sound /m/ at the beginning of 'move.' "
- "mouse (*pause*) Yes, I hear the sound /m/ at the beginning of 'mouse.' "
- "nose (*pause*) No, I don't hear the sound /m/ at the beginning of 'nose.' "
- "math (*pause*) Yes, I hear /m/ at the beginning of 'math.' "
- "sleepy (*pause*) No, I don't hear /m/ at the beginning of 'sleepy.' "
- "book (*pause*) No, I don't hear /m/ at the beginning of 'book.' "
- "marbles (*pause*) Yes, I hear /m/ at the beginning of 'marbles.' "

Listening and Looking for /m/ in the Beginning, Middle, or End of Words

- "Now all the words I say are going to have the sound /m/ in the word, but you have to listen very carefully and watch my mouth as I say the words. When I call on someone, your job will be to tell me if you heard the sound /m/ at the beginning (first sound), middle, or end (last sound) of the word. For example, if I say the word 'farm,' the /m/ sound is at the end of the word. 'Farm'—hear the /m/ at the end? If I say 'milk,' the /m/ sound is the beginning sound in the word."
- climb (end)
- name (end)
- money (beginning)
- thumb (end)
- magnet (beginning)
- women (middle)
- major (beginning)
- some (end)
- cream (end)
- mirror (beginning)
- family (middle)
- mystery (beginning)

Phoneme /n/ (Letter *n*)

Information for the Teacher

- Place: tongue up on ridge behind front top teeth (alveolar ridge)
- Voicing: voice on (voiced)
- Manner: air passes through the nose (nasal)
- Common spellings: *n*-nose, *gn*-gnat, *kn*-know, *nn*-dinner, *pn*-pneumonia

Information for the Children

- "Today we are talking about the /n/ sound. There is one letter that most often makes the /n/ sound, the letter *n*."
- "I make the /n/ by placing the tip of my tongue behind my front top teeth. When I blow the air it comes out of my nose, and I can hear my voice when I say the /n/ sound."
- "Listen and watch my mouth as I make the /n/ sound: /nnnnnnnnnn/." (Draw the sound out as you say it.)
- "Now you practice saying the /n/ sound several times. Feel your tongue touch the bumpy part behind your teeth as you say it. I'll hand out some mirrors to pass around. Look in the mirror as you say /n/ two times, then pass the mirror to the next child."

Listening and Looking for the /n/ Sound by Itself

- "Nod your head yes if you hear the /n/ sound. Shake your head no if you don't hear the /n/ sound."
- "/n/ (*pause*) Yes, that was the /n/ sound."
- "/s/ (*pause*) No, that was not the /n/ sound."
- "/k/ (*pause*) No, that was not the /n/ sound."
- "/n/ (*pause*) Yes, that was the /n/ sound."
- "/g/ (*pause*) No, that was not the /n/ sound."
- "/d/ (*pause*) That is a hard one. It's not the /n/ sound. We make the /d/ sound with our tongue in the same place as the /n/ sound, but the /d/ sound is a short sound and air blows out of our mouth. The /n/ is a long sound and air comes out of our nose. Listen again to the difference between /d/ and /n/: /d/ is short and /n/ is long."
- "/f/ (*pause*) No, that was not the /n/ sound."
- "/n/ (*pause*) Yes, that was the /n/ sound."
- "/m/ (*pause*) No, that was not the /n/ sound." (If any children have nodded their heads indicating that it was the /n/ sound, explain that /m/ is a loud sound that blows air out of the nose like the /n/ sound but the /n/ sound is different because the front tip of the tongue goes up behind the front teeth instead of the lips coming together for /m/. Compare /n/ and /m/ again, with special attention to how the mouth and lips move. Open your mouth a little more for the /n/

to let the children see where the tongue is placed for the /n/ sound. Ask the children to repeat /m/ and /n/ and to feel how their tongues and lips move differently for the two sounds.)

Listening and Looking for /n/ in the Beginning of Words

- "Now we're going to listen for the /n/ sound in words. Nod your head yes if /n/ is the first sound in the word I say. Shake your head no if you don't hear /n/ at the beginning of the word."
- "new (*pause*) Yes, I hear the sound /n/ at the beginning of 'new.'"
- "night (*pause*) Yes, I hear the sound /n/ at the beginning of 'night.'"
- "place (*pause*) No, I don't hear the sound /n/ at the beginning of 'place.'"
- "north (*pause*) Yes, I hear /n/ at the beginning of 'north.'"
- "more (*pause*) No, I don't hear /n/ at the beginning of 'more.'"
- "big (*pause*) No, I don't hear /n/ at the beginning of 'big.'"
- "knife (*pause*) Yes, I hear /n/ at the beginning of 'knife.'"

Listening and Looking for /n/ in the Beginning, Middle, or End of Words

- "Now all the words I say are going to have the sound /n/ in the word, but you have to listen very carefully and watch my mouth as I say the words. When I call on you, your job will be to tell me if you heard the sound /n/ at the beginning (first sound), middle, or end (last sound) of the word. For example, if I say the word 'fan,' the /n/ sound is at the end of the word. 'Fan'— hear the /n/ at the end? If I say 'nurse,' the /n/ sound is the beginning sound in the word."
- win (end)
- yawn (end)
- nap (beginning)
- skin (end)
- near (beginning)
- planet (middle)
- nice (beginning)
- coin (end)
- crown (end)
- noodle (beginning)
- canoe (middle)
- nothing (beginning)

Phoneme /p/ (Letter *p*)

Information for the Teacher

- Place: both lips (bilabial)
- Voicing: quiet (voiceless)
- Manner: stop (air blocked, then blown out)
- Common spellings: *p*-pull, *pp*-happy, *ph*-shepherd

Information for the Children

- "Today we are talking about the /p/ sound. There is one letter that most often makes the /p/ sound, the letter *p*."
- "I make the /p/ by putting my lips together. When my lips come apart quickly, the air blows out and I do not hear my voice when I say it."
- "Listen and watch my mouth as I make the /p/ sound: /p/, /p/, /p/, /p/, /p/, /p/." (Move your lips apart and then together when making the /p/ sound to exaggerate the movement of the lips.)
- "Now you practice saying the /p/ sound several times. Feel your lips touch together and come apart as you say it. You can put your hand in front of your mouth and feel the air puff out as you say it. The /p/ sound is a quiet sound. I just hear air puffing—my voice isn't turned on. I'll hand out some mirrors to pass around. Look in the mirror as you say /p/ two times, then pass the mirror to the next child."

Listening and Looking for the /p/ Sound by Itself

- "Nod your head yes if you see and hear the /p/ sound. Shake your head no if you don't hear the /p/ sound."
- "/p/ (*pause*) Yes, that was the /p/ sound."
- "/s/ (*pause*) No, that was not the /p/ sound."
- "/n/ (*pause*) No, that was not the /p/ sound."
- "/p/ (*pause*) Yes, that was the /p/ sound."
- "/k/ (*pause*) No, that was not the /p/ sound."
- "/b/ (*pause*) That is a hard one. It's not the /p/ sound. We make the /b/ sound somewhat like the /p/ sound, but the /p/ sound is a quiet sound. We have our voice off when we say the /p/ sound, but the /b/ is a loud sound with our voice on. Listen again to the difference between /b/ and /p/: /p/ is quiet; /b/ is louder with our voice on."
- "/f/ (*pause*) No, that was not the /p/ sound."
- "/p/ (*pause*) Yes, that was the /p/ sound."
- "/t/ (*pause*) No, that was not the /p/ sound." (If any children have nodded their heads indicating that it was the /p/ sound, explain that /t/ is a quiet sound that blows air out like the /p/ sound but the /t/ sound is different because the front tip of the tongue goes up behind the front teeth instead of the lips coming together. Compare /p/ and /t/ again, with special atten-

tion to how the mouth and lips move. Open your mouth a little more for the /t/ to let the children see where the tongue and lips are placed for the /t/ and /p/ sounds. Ask the children to repeat /p/ and /t/ and to feel how their tongues and lips move differently for the two sounds.)

Listening and Looking for /p/ in the Beginning of Words

- "Now we're going to listen for the /p/ sound in words. Nod your head yes if /p/ is the first sound in the word I say. Shake your head no if you don't hear /p/ at the beginning of the word."
- "paint (*pause*) Yes, I hear the sound /p/ at the beginning of 'paint.'"
- "pink (*pause*) Yes, I hear the sound /p/ at the beginning of 'pink.'"
- "door (*pause*) No, I don't hear the sound /p/ at the beginning of 'door.'"
- "pound (*pause*) Yes, I hear /p/ at the beginning of 'pound.'"
- "bounce (*pause*) No, I don't hear /p/ at the beginning of 'bounce.'" (If there is any confusion, have the class listen to the word "pounce" with /p/ emphasized at the beginning and "bounce" with /b/ emphasized at the beginning.)
- "short (*pause*) No, I don't hear /p/ at the beginning of 'short.'"
- "package (*pause*) Yes, I hear /p/ at the beginning of 'package.'"

Listening and Looking for /p/ in the Beginning, Middle, or End of Words

- "Now all the words I say are going to have the sound /p/ in the word, but you have to listen very carefully and watch my mouth as I say the words. When I call on someone, your job will be to tell me if you heard the sound /p/ at the beginning (first sound), middle, or end (last sound) of the word. For example, if I say the word 'cup,' the /p/ sound is at the end of the word. 'Cup'—hear the /p/ at the end? If I say 'pull,' the /p/ sound is the beginning sound in the word."
- clap (end)
- help (end)
- pencil (beginning)
- soup (end)
- power (beginning)
- shopper (middle)
- poison (beginning)
- hop (end)
- soap (end)
- police (beginning)
- repeat (middle)
- patient (beginning)

Phoneme /r/ (Letter *r*)

Information for the Teacher

- Place: tongue bunched up high in the middle of mouth (palatal)
- Voicing: voice on (voiced)
- Manner: liquid
- Common spellings: *r*-red, *wr*-write, *rr*-carrot, *rh*-rhyme

Information for the Children

- "Today we are talking about the /r/ sound. The letter *r* makes the /r/ sound."
- "/r/ is a sound like a lion roaring." (Make an *r*-like roaring /rrrrr-rrrrrr/. Ask children to make an *r*-roar too.)
- "I make the /r/ by bunching up my tongue in the middle of my mouth. The /r/ sound is a loud sound—I hear my voice on when I say /r/."
- "Listen and watch my mouth as I make the /r/ sound, /r/, /r/, /r/, /r/, /r/, /r/."
- "Now you practice saying the /r/ sound several times. Feel where your tongue is bunched up and tight in the middle of your mouth. Feel how you turn on your voice and keep your tongue bunched up tight as you say /r/. I'll hand out some mirrors to pass around. Look in the mirror as you say /r/ two times, then pass the mirror to the next child."

Listening and Looking for the /r/ Sound by Itself

- "Watch my mouth and listen carefully as I say some sounds. Nod your head yes if you hear the /r/ sound. Shake your head no if you don't hear the /r/ sound."
- "/r/ (*pause*) Yes, that was the /r/ sound."
- "/l/ (*pause*) No, that was not the /r/ sound."
- "/w/ (*pause*) No, that was not the /r/ sound." (If any children have nodded their heads indicating that it was the /r/ sound, explain that /w/ is a loud sound like /r/ but the /w/ sound is different because we pucker up and move our lips to say /w/ whereas for /r/ we leave our lips still and just bunch up our tongue tight in the middle of our mouth. Compare /w/ and /r/ again. Ask the children to repeat /w/ and /r/ and to feel how their mouths move differently for the two sounds.)
- "/r/ (*pause*) Yes, that was the /r/ sound."
- "/n/ (*pause*) No, that was not the /r/ sound."
- "/r/ (*pause*) Yes, that was the /r/ sound."
- "/l/ (*pause*) No, that was not the /r/ sound."
- "/m/ (*pause*) No, that was not the /r/ sound."
- "/g/ (*pause*) No, that was not the /r/ sound."
- "/r/ (*pause*) Yes, that was the /r/ sound."

Listening and Looking for /r/ in the Beginning of Words

- "Now we're going to listen and look for the /r/ sound in words. Watch my mouth as I say these words. Nod your head yes if /r/ is the first sound in the word I say. Shake your head no if you don't hear /r/ at the beginning of the word."
- "red (*pause*) Yes, I hear the sound /r/ at the beginning of 'red.'"
- "rake (*pause*) Yes, I hear the sound /r/ at the beginning of 'rake.'"
- "window (*pause*) No, I don't hear the sound /r/ at the beginning of 'window.'"
- "rain (*pause*) Yes, I hear /r/ at the beginning of 'rain.'"
- "light (*pause*) No, I don't hear /r/ at the beginning of 'light.'"
- "juice (*pause*) No, I don't hear /r/ at the beginning of 'juice.'"
- "rainbow (*pause*) Yes, I hear /r/ at the beginning of 'rainbow.'"

Listening and Looking for /r/ in the Beginning, Middle, or End of Words

- "Now all of the words I say are going to have the sound /r/ in the word, but you have to listen very carefully and watch my mouth as I say the words. When I call on you, your job will be to tell me if you heard the sound /r/ at the beginning (first sound), middle, or end (last sound) of the word. For example, if I say the word 'bear,' the /r/ sound is at the end of the word. 'Bear,' hear /r/ at the end? If I say 'rope,' the /r/ sound is the beginning sound in the word."
- race (beginning)
- chair (end)
- flower (end)
- story (middle)
- hour (end)
- read (beginning)
- carrot (middle)
- reach (beginning)
- right (beginning)
- fire (end)
- hair (end)

Phoneme /s/ (Letter *s*)

Information for the Teacher

- Place: tongue near ridge behind front top teeth (alveolar ridge)
- Voicing: quiet (voiceless)
- Manner: fricative (noisy air continuously blowing out)
- Common spellings: *s*-soup, *ss*-kiss, *c*-piece, *sc*-scissors, *z*-waltz

Information for the Children

- "Today we are talking about the /s/ sound. The letter *s* makes the /s/ sound, but the letter *c* also makes the /s/ sound sometimes."
- "I make the /s/ with the front part of my tongue behind my top teeth and blowing air out. The /s/ sound is a quiet sound. I just hear air blowing—I don't hear my voice on when I say it."
- "/s/ is the sound that snakes make."
- "Listen and watch my mouth as I make the /s/ sound: /sssssssssssssss/." (Draw the sound out as you say it.)
- "Now you practice saying the /s/ (snake) sound several times. Feel your tongue move just behind your top front teeth. I'll hand out some mirrors to pass around. Look in the mirror as you say /s/ two times, then pass the mirror to the next child."

Listening and Looking for the /s/ Sound by Itself

- "Watch my mouth and listen carefully as I say some sounds. Nod your head yes if you hear and see the /s/ sound. Shake your head no if you don't hear the /s/ sound."
- "/s/ (*pause*) Yes, that was the /s/ sound."
- "/r/ (*pause*) No, that was not the /s/ sound."
- "/m/ (*pause*) No, that was not the /s/ sound."
- "/s/ (*pause*) Yes, that was the /s/ sound."
- "/z/ (*pause*) That is a hard one. It's not the /s/ sound. We make the /z/ sound somewhat like the /s/ sound, but the /z/ sound is a loud sound. We have our voice on when we say the /z/ sound, but /s/ is a quiet sound with our voice off. Listen again to the difference between /s/ and /z/: /s/ is quiet; /z/ is louder, with our voice on."
- "/k/ (*pause*) No, that was not the /s/ sound."
- "/s/ (*pause*) Yes, that was the /s/ sound."
- "/f/ (*pause*) No, that was not the /s/ sound." (If any children have nodded their heads indicating that it was the /s/ sound, explain that /f/ is a quiet sound that blows air out like the /s/ sound but the /s/ sound is different because the front tip of the tongue goes up behind the front teeth instead of the top teeth touching the bottom lip for /f/. Compare /s/ and /f/ again, pointing to your mouth as you say the sounds so that the children can see the difference in

what moves as you say those sounds. Ask the children to repeat /s/ and /f/ and to feel how their mouths move differently for the two sounds.)

Listening and Looking for /s/ in the Beginning of Words

- "Now we're going to listen and look for the /s/ sound in words. Watch my mouth as I say these words. Nod your head yes if /s/ is the first sound in the word I say. Shake your head no if you don't hear /s/ at the beginning of the word."
- "sing (*pause*) Yes, I hear the sound /s/ at the beginning of 'sing.' "
- "sit (*pause*) Yes, I hear the sound /s/ at the beginning of 'sit.' "
- "fight (*pause*) No, I don't hear the sound /s/ at the beginning of 'fight.' "
- "Sunday (*pause*) Yes, I hear /s/ at the beginning of 'Sunday.' "
- "chair (*pause*) No, I don't hear /s/ at the beginning of 'chair.' "
- "brother (*pause*) No, I don't hear /s/ at the beginning of 'brother.' "
- "sale (*pause*) Yes, I hear /s/ at the beginning of 'sale.' "

Listening and Looking for /s/ in the Beginning, Middle, or End of Words

- "Now all the words I say are going to have the sound /s/ in the word, but you have to listen very carefully and watch my mouth as I say the words. When I call on you, your job will be to tell me if you heard the sound /s/ at the beginning (first sound), middle, or end (last sound) of the word. For example, if I say the word 'grass,' the /s/ sound is at the end of the word. 'Grass'—hear the /s/ at the end? If I say 'sick,' the /s/ sound is the beginning sound in the word."
- icy (middle)
- guess (end)
- same (beginning)
- castle (middle)
- sour (beginning)
- mouse (end)
- jealous (end)
- hospital (middle)
- sailor (beginning)
- whistle (middle)
- saving (beginning)

Phoneme /t/ (Letter *t*)

Information for the Teacher

- Place: tongue on ridge behind front top teeth (alveolar ridge)
- Voicing: quiet (voiceless)
- Manner: stop (air blocked, then blown out)
- Common spellings: *t*-tap, *tt*-little, *bt*-debt, *d*-hoped, *pt*-receipt

Information for the Children

- "Today we are talking about the /t/ sound. There is one letter that often makes the /t/ sound, the letter *t*."
- "I make the /t/ with the front of my tongue touching the place behind my top front teeth. When my tongue tip drops down a little, the air blows out. The /t/ sound is a quiet sound. I just hear air blowing—I don't hear my voice on when I say it."
- "Listen and watch my mouth as I make the /t/ sound: /t/, /t/, /t/, /t/, /t/, /t/, /t/." (Open your mouth a little wider than usual for a couple of /t/ productions so that the children see the front of your tongue moving up and down as you say the sound.)
- "Now you practice saying the /t/ sound several times. Feel how your tongue goes up behind your teeth and then air blows out as you say it. Don't turn your voice on. The /t/ sound is a quiet sound. You should just hear air blowing. I'll hand out some mirrors to pass around. Look in the mirror as you say /t/ two times, then pass the mirror to the next child."

Listening and Looking for the /t/ Sound by Itself

- "Nod your head yes if you hear the /t/ sound. Shake your head no if you don't hear the /t/ sound."
- "/t/ (*pause*) Yes, that was the /t/ sound."
- "/s/ (*pause*) No, that was not the /t/ sound."
- "/m/ (*pause*) No, that was not the /t/ sound."
- "/t/ (*pause*) Yes, that was the /t/ sound."
- "/d/ (*pause*) That is a hard one. It's not the /t/ sound. We make the /d/ sound somewhat like the /t/ sound, but the /d/ sound is a loud sound. We have our voice on when we say the /d/ sound, but the /t/ is a quiet sound with our voice off. Listen again to the difference between /t/ and /d/: the /t/ is quiet, the /d/ is louder with our voice on."
- "/f/ (*pause*) No, that was not the /t/ sound."
- "/t/ (*pause*) Yes, that was the /t/ sound."
- "/k/ (*pause*) No, that was not the /t/ sound." (If any children have nodded their heads indicating that it was the /t/ sound, explain that /k/ is a quiet sound that blows air out like the /t/ sound but the /k/ sound is different because the back of tongue goes up for /k/ and the front tip of the tongue goes up behind the front teeth for /t/. Compare /t/ and /k/ again with your

mouth slightly more open than usual so that the children can see the different ways in which part of your tongue moves as you say those sounds. Ask the children to repeat /t/ and /k/ and feel how their tongues move differently for the two sounds.)

Listening and Looking for /t/ in the Beginning of Words

- "Now we're going to listen for the /t/ sound in words. Nod your head yes if /t/ is the first sound in the word I say. Shake your head no if you don't hear /t/ at the beginning of the word."
- "tall (*pause*) Yes, I hear the sound /t/ at the beginning of 'tall.' "
- "toe (*pause*) Yes, I hear the sound /t/ at the beginning of 'toe.' "
- "move (*pause*) No, I don't hear the sound /t/ at the beginning of 'move.' "
- "tiny (*pause*) Yes, I hear /t/ at the beginning of 'tiny.' "
- "fish (*pause*) No, I don't hear /t/ at the beginning of 'fish.' "
- "cool (*pause*) No, I don't hear /t/ at the beginning of 'cool.' "
- "tangle (*pause*) Yes, I hear /t/ at the beginning of 'tangle.' "

Listening and Looking for /t/ in the Beginning, Middle, or End of Words

- "Now all the words I say are going to have the sound /t/ in the word, but you have to listen very carefully and watch my mouth as I say the words. When I call on you, your job will be to tell me if you heard the sound /t/ at the beginning (first sound), middle, or end (last sound) of the word. For example, if I say the word 'hat,' the /t/ sound is at the end of the word. 'Hat'—hear the /t/ at the end? If I say 'table,' the /t/ sound is the beginning sound in the word."
- boat (end)
- feet (end)
- toss (beginning)
- fight (end)
- telephone (beginning)
- hotdog (middle)
- batting (middle)
- tornado (beginning)
- rabbit (end)
- forget (end)
- teach (beginning)
- dirty (middle)
- water (middle)
- time (beginning)

Phoneme /v/ (Letter *v*)

Information for the Teacher

- Place: top teeth on bottom lip (dental)
- Voicing: voice on (voiced)
- Manner: fricative (noisy air continuously blowing out)
- Common spellings: *v*-van, *f*-of, *ph*-Stephen

Information for the Children

- "Today we are talking about the /v/ sound. The letter *v* makes the /v/ sound."
- "I make the /v/ with my top teeth touching my bottom lip, turning on my voice and blowing air out. The /v/ sound is a loud sound. I hear my voice on when I say it."
- "Listen and watch my mouth as I make the /v/ sound: /v/, /v/, /v/, /v/, /v/, /v/."
- "Now you practice saying the /v/ sound several times. Feel where your top teeth touch your bottom lip as you say /v/. Feel your neck and throat to feel your voice turned on as you say /v/. I'll hand out some mirrors to pass around. Look in the mirror as you say /v/ two times, then pass the mirror to the next child."

Listening and Looking for the /v/ Sound by Itself

- "Watch my mouth and listen carefully as I say some sounds. Nod your head yes if you hear and see the /v/ sound. Shake your head no if you don't hear the /v/ sound."
- "/v/ (*pause*) Yes, that was the /v/ sound."
- "/w/ (*pause*) No, that was not the /v/ sound."
- "/l/ (*pause*) No, that was not the /v/ sound."
- "/v/ (*pause*) Yes, that was the /v/ sound."
- "/f/ (*pause*) That is a hard one. It's not the /v/ sound. We make the /f/ sound somewhat like the /v/ sound, but the /v/ sound is a loud sound. We have our voice on when we say the /v/ sound, but /f/ is a quiet sound with our voice off. Listen again to the difference between /f/ and /v/: the /f/ is quiet; the /v/ sound is louder with our voice on."
- "/g/ (*pause*) No, that was not the /v/ sound."
- "/v/ (*pause*) Yes, that was the /v/ sound."
- "/z/ (*pause*) No, that was not the /v/ sound." (If any children have nodded their heads indicating that it was the /z/ sound, explain that /z/ is a loud sound that blows air out like the /v/ sound but the /z/ sound is different because the front tip of the tongue goes up behind the front teeth instead of the top teeth touching the bottom lip for /v/. Compare /z/ and /v/ again, pointing to your mouth as you say the sounds so that the children can see the difference in what moves as you say those sounds. Ask the children to repeat /z/ and /v/ and to feel how their mouths move differently for the two sounds.)

Listening and Looking for /v/ at the Beginning of Words

- "Now we're going to listen and look for the /v/ sound in words. Watch my mouth as I say these words. Nod your head yes if /v/ is the first sound in the word I say. Shake your head no if you don't hear /v/ at the beginning of the word."
- "visit (*pause*) Yes, I hear the sound /v/ at the beginning of 'visit.'"
- "vacuum (*pause*) Yes, I hear the sound /v/ at the beginning of 'vacuum.'"
- "zebra (*pause*) No, I don't hear the sound /v/ at the beginning of 'zebra.'"
- "valentine (*pause*) Yes, I hear /v/ at the beginning of 'valentine.'"
- "shake (*pause*) No, I don't hear /v/ at the beginning of 'shake.'"
- "that (*pause*) No, I don't hear /v/ at the beginning of 'that.'"
- "van (*pause*) Yes, I hear /v/ at the beginning of 'van.'"

Listening and Looking for /v/ in the Beginning, Middle, or End of Words

- "Now all the words I say are going to have the sound /v/ in the word, but you have to listen very carefully and watch my mouth as I say the words. When I call on someone, your job will be to tell me if you heard the sound /v/ at the beginning (first sound), middle, or end (last sound) of the word. For example, if I say the word 'love,' the /v/ sound is at the end of the word. 'Love'—hear the /v/ at the end? If I say 'vote,' the /v/ sound is the beginning sound in the word."
- volleyball (beginning)
- dive (end)
- glove (end)
- event (middle)
- vase (beginning)
- over (middle)
- visit (beginning)
- move (end)
- travel (middle)
- believe (end)
- vine (beginning)
- oven (middle)

Phoneme /w/ (Letter *w*)

Information for the Teacher

- Place: two lips (bilabial)
- Voicing: voice on (voiced)
- Manner: glide (lips move from puckered to unpuckered during /w/ production)
- Common spellings: *w*-water, *wh*-what
- /w/ only occurs at the beginning and middle of words.

Information for the Children

- "Today we are talking about the /w/ sound. The letter *w* makes the /w/ sound."
- "I make the /w/ by puckering up my lips a little bit. The /w/ sound is a loud sound. I hear my voice on when I say /w/."
- "Listen and watch my mouth as I make the /w/ sound: /w/, /w/, /w/, /w/, /w/."
- "Now you practice saying the /w/ sound several times. Feel how your lips move and pucker up and your voice is turned on as you say /w/. I'll hand out some mirrors to pass around. Look in the mirror as you say /w/ two times, then pass the mirror to the next child."

Listening and Looking for the /w/ Sound by Itself

- "Watch my mouth and listen carefully as I say some sounds. Nod your head yes if you hear the /w/ sound. Shake your head no if you don't hear the /w/ sound."
- "/w/ (*pause*) Yes, that was the /w/ sound."
- "/l/ (*pause*) No, that was not the /w/ sound."
- "/r/ (*pause*) No, that was not the /w/ sound." (If any children have nodded their heads indicating that it was the /w/ sound, explain that /w/ is a loud sound like /r/ but the /w/ sound is different because we pucker up and move our lips to say /w/ whereas for /r/ we bunch up our tongue tight in the middle of our mouth. Compare /w/ and /r/ again. Ask the children to repeat /w/ and /r/ and to feel how their mouths move differently for the two sounds.)
- "/w/ (*pause*) Yes, that was the /w/ sound."
- "/b/ (*pause*) No, that was not the /w/ sound." (If any children have nodded their heads indicating that it was the /w/ sound, explain that we move the lips, put them together, and blow air out for /b/, but we pucker the lips to make /w/.)
- "/w/ (*pause*) Yes, that was the /w/ sound."
- "/n/ (*pause*) No, that was not the /w/ sound."
- "/g/ (*pause*) No, that was not the /w/ sound."
- "/w/ (*pause*) Yes, that was the /w/ sound."

Listening and Looking for /w/ at the Beginning of Words

- "Now we're going to listen and look for the /w/ sound in words. Watch my mouth as I say these words. Nod your head yes if /w/ is the first sound in the word I say. Shake your head no if you don't hear /w/ at the beginning of the word."
- "water (*pause*) Yes, I hear the sound /w/ at the beginning of 'water.'"
- "wide (*pause*) Yes, I hear the sound /w/ at the beginning of 'wide.'"
- "milk (*pause*) No, I don't hear the sound /w/ at the beginning of 'milk.'"
- "wedding (*pause*) Yes, I hear /w/ at the beginning of 'wedding.'"
- "lake (*pause*) No, I don't hear /w/ at the beginning of 'lake.'"
- "rain (*pause*) No, I don't hear /w/ at the beginning of 'rain.'"
- "why (*pause*) Yes, I hear /w/ at the beginning of 'why.'"

Listening and Looking for /w/ in the Beginning and Middle of Words

- "Now all of the words I say are going to have the sound /w/ in the word, but you have to listen very carefully and watch my mouth as I say the words. When I call on you, your job will be to tell me if you heard the sound /w/ at the beginning (first sound) or middle of the word. For example, if I say 'when,' the /w/ sound is the beginning sound of the word."
- wall (beginning)
- flower (middle)
- word (beginning)
- always (middle)
- want (beginning)
- somewhere (middle)
- wheel (beginning)
- weather (beginning)

Phoneme /j/ (Letter *y*)

Information for the Teacher

- Place: tongue arched in the middle of mouth (palatal)
- Voicing: voice on (voiced)
- Manner: glide (tongue arches then glides slightly lower during /j/ production)
- Common spellings: *y*-yellow. (*Note:* The /j/ sound does not occur at the end of words in English. The /j/ sound is in the middle of many words without a consonant to represent the sound. For example, "onion"—/j/ in the middle after the first *n*; "few"—/j/ sound after *f*; "Daniel"—/j/ sound after *n*; "union"—/j/ sound in the middle after the first *n*. Because /j/ does not occur at the end of words and is not often represented with a *consonant* in the middle of words, a section on listening for /j/ in the beginning, middle, or end of words is not included for this sound.)

Information for the Children

- "Today we are talking about the /j/ sound. The letter *y* makes the /j/ sound."
- "I make the /j/ sound by arching up my tongue in the middle of my mouth. The /j/ sound is a loud sound. I hear my voice on when I say /j/."
- "Listen and watch my mouth as I make the /j/ sound: /j/, /j/, /j/, /j/, /j/, /j/, /j/."
- "Now you practice saying the /j/ sound several times. Feel where your tongue is in the middle of your mouth. Feel how you turn on your voice and move your tongue down a little bit in the middle of your mouth as you say /j/. I'll hand out some mirrors to pass around. Look in the mirror as you say /j/ two times, then pass the mirror to the next child."

Listening and Looking for the /j/ Sound by Itself

- "Watch my mouth and listen carefully as I say some sounds. Nod your head yes if you hear the /j/ sound. Shake your head no if you don't hear the /j/ sound."
- "/j/ (*pause*) Yes, that was the /j/ sound."
- "/w/ (*pause*) No, that was not the /j/ sound." (If any children have nodded their heads indicating that it was the /j/ sound, explain that /w/ is a loud sound like /j/ but the /w/ sound is different because we pucker up and move our lips to say /w/ whereas for /j/ we leave our lips still and just arch up our tongue in the middle of our mouth. Compare /w/ and /j/ again. Ask the children to repeat /w/ and /j/ and to feel how their mouths move differently for the two sounds.)
- "/j/ (*pause*) Yes, that was the /j/ sound."
- "/n/ (*pause*) No, that was not the /j/ sound."
- "/j/ (*pause*) Yes, that was the /j/ sound."
- "/l/ (*pause*) No, that was not the /j/ sound." (If any children have nodded their heads indicating that it was the /j/ sound, explain that /l/ is a loud sound like /j/ but the /l/ sound is different

because we touch our tongue on the ridge behind the teeth for /l/ whereas for /j/ we just arch up our tongue in the middle of our mouth. Compare /l/ and /j/ again. Ask the children to repeat /l/ and /j/ and to feel how their mouths move differently for the two sounds.)

- "/j/ (*pause*) Yes, that was the /j/ sound."
- "/m/ (*pause*) No, that was not the /j/ sound."
- "/g/ (*pause*) No, that was not the /j/ sound."
- "/j/ (*pause*) Yes, that was the /j/ sound."

Listening and Looking for /j/ at the Beginning of Words

- "Now we're going to listen and look for the /j/ sound in words. Watch my mouth as I say these words. Nod your head yes if /j/ is the first sound in the word I say. Shake your head no if you don't hear /j/ at the beginning of the word."
- "yellow (*pause*) Yes, I hear the sound /j/ at the beginning of 'yellow.'"
- "you (*pause*) Yes, I hear the sound /j/ at the beginning of 'you.'"
- "walk (*pause*) No, I don't hear the sound /j/ at the beginning of 'walk.'"
- "yell (*pause*) Yes, I hear /j/ at the beginning of 'yell.'"
- "light (*pause*) No, I don't hear /j/ at the beginning of 'light.'"
- "mom (*pause*) No, I don't hear /j/ at the beginning of 'mom.'"
- "young (*pause*) Yes, I hear /j/ at the beginning of 'young.'"
- "yo-yo (*pause*) Yes, I hear /j/ at the beginning (as well as the middle) of 'yo-yo.'"

Phoneme /z/ (Letter z)

Information for the Teacher

- Place: tongue near the ridge behind front top teeth (alveolar ridge)
- Voicing: voice on (voiced)
- Manner: fricative (noisy air continuously blowing out)
- Common spellings: *z*-zebra, *zz*-buzz, *s*-shoes

Information for the Children

- "Today we are talking about the /z/ sound. The letter *z* makes the /z/ sound, but the letter *s* also makes the /z/ sound sometimes."
- "I make the /z/ with the front part of my tongue behind my top teeth and blowing air out. The /z/ sound is a loud sound because I turn on my voice when I say it."
- "Listen and watch my mouth as I make the /z/ sound: /z/, /z/, /z/, /z/, /z/, /z/, /z/."
- "Now you practice saying the /z/ sound several times. Feel your tongue move just behind your top front teeth. Feel how your voice is on and air blows out the whole time you say /z/. I'll hand out some mirrors to pass around. Look in the mirror as you say /z/ two times, then pass the mirror to the next child."

Listening and Looking for the /z/ Sound by Itself

- "Watch my mouth and listen carefully as I say some sounds. Nod your head yes if you hear and see the /z/ sound. Shake your head no if you don't hear the /z/ sound."
- "/z/ (*pause*) Yes, that was the /z/ sound."
- "/r/ (*pause*) No, that was not the /z/ sound."
- "/n/ (*pause*) No, that was not the /z/ sound."
- "/z/ (*pause*) Yes, that was the /z/ sound."
- "/s/ (*pause*) That is a hard one. It's not the /z/ sound. We make the /s/ sound somewhat like the /z/ sound, but the /s/ sound is a quiet sound. We have our voice on when we say the /z/ sound, but /s/ is a quiet sound with our voice off. Listen again to the difference between /s/ and /z/: /s/ is quiet; the /z/ sound is louder with our voice on."
- "/k/ (*pause*) No, that was not the /z/ sound."
- "/z/ (*pause*) Yes, that was the /z/ sound."
- "/v/ (*pause*) No, that was not the /z/ sound." (If any children nod their heads indicating that it was the /z/ sound, explain that /z/ is a loud sound that blows air out like the /v/ sound but the /z/ sound is different because the front tip of the tongue goes up behind the front teeth instead of the top teeth touching the bottom lip for /v/. Compare /z/ and /v/ again, pointing to your mouth as you say the sounds so that the children can see the difference in what moves as you say those sounds. Ask the children to repeat /z/ and /v/ and to feel how their mouth moves differently for the two sounds.)

Listening and Looking for /z/ at the Beginning of Words

- "Now we're going to listen and look for the /z/ sound in words. Watch my mouth as I say these words. Nod your head yes if /z/ is the first sound in the word I say. Shake your head no if you don't hear /z/ at the beginning of the word."
- "zoo (*pause*) Yes, I hear the sound /z/ at the beginning of 'zoo.'"
- "zap (*pause*) Yes, I hear the sound /z/ at the beginning of 'zap.'"
- "van (*pause*) No, I don't hear the sound /z/ at the beginning of 'van.'"
- "zebra (*pause*) Yes, I hear /z/ at the beginning of 'zebra.'"
- "sleeve (*pause*) No, I don't hear /z/ at the beginning of 'sleeve.'"
- "feather (*pause*) No, I don't hear /z/ at the beginning of 'feather.'"
- "zipper (*pause*) Yes, I hear /z/ at the beginning of 'zipper.'"

Listening and Looking for /z/ in the Beginning, Middle, or End of Words

- "Now all the words I say are going to have the sound /z/ in the word, but you have to listen very carefully and watch my mouth as I say the words. When I call on someone, your job will be to tell me if you heard the sound /z/ at the beginning (first sound), middle, or end (last sound) of the word. For example, if I say the word 'buzz,' the /z/ sound is at the end of the word. 'Buzz'—hear the /z/ at the end? If I say 'zoom,' the /z/ sound is the beginning sound in the word."
- puzzle (middle)
- freeze (end)
- pleasant (middle)
- zero (beginning)
- noise (end)
- news (end)
- visit (middle)
- zip (beginning)
- dizzy (middle)
- Zachary (beginning)
- clothes (end)

Phoneme /ʃ/ (Digraph *sh*)

Information for the Teacher

- Place: tongue in the middle of mouth (palatal)
- Voicing: quiet (voiceless)
- Manner: fricative (noisy air continuously blowing out)
- Common spellings: *sh*-shoe, *ti*-nation/patient, *c*-special/ocean, *ch*-machine, *s*-sugar, *ss*-mission

Information for the Children

- "Today we are talking about the /ʃ/ sound. The letters *sh* make the /ʃ/ sound."
- "The /ʃ/ sound is the sound we make when we want someone to be quiet." (Put your finger up to your mouth and say /ʃ/.)
- "I make the /ʃ/ with my tongue back in the middle of my mouth and blowing air out. Sometimes my lips pucker a little bit when I say /ʃ/. The /ʃ/ sound is a quiet sound. I just hear air blowing—I don't hear my voice on when I say it."
- "Listen and watch my mouth as I make the /ʃ/ sound: /ʃ/, /ʃ/, /ʃ/, /ʃ/, /ʃ/, /ʃ/."
- "Now you practice saying the /ʃ/ sound several times. Feel where your tongue is in the middle of your mouth and your lips may pucker a little bit as you say /ʃ/ and air blows out. I'll hand out some mirrors to pass around. Look in the mirror as you say /ʃ/ two times, then pass the mirror to the next child."

Listening and Looking for the /ʃ/ Sound by Itself

- "Watch my mouth and listen carefully as I say some sounds. Nod your head yes if you hear and see the /ʃ/ sound. Shake your head no if you don't hear the /ʃ/ sound."
- "/ʃ/ (*pause*) Yes, that was the /ʃ/ sound."
- "/f/ (*pause*) No, that was not the /ʃ/ sound."
- "/m/ (*pause*) No, that was not the /ʃ/ sound."
- "/ʃ/ (*pause*) Yes, that was the /ʃ/ sound."
- "/k/ (*pause*) No, that was not the /ʃ/ sound."
- "/ʃ/ (*pause*) Yes, that was the /ʃ/ sound."
- "/s/ (*pause*) No, that was not the /ʃ/ sound." (If any children have nodded their heads indicating that it was the /ʃ/ sound, explain that /s/ is a quiet sound that blows air out like the /ʃ/ sound but the /s/ sound is different because the front tip of the tongue goes up behind the front teeth instead of the middle of the tongue for /ʃ/, with lips possibly puckering. Compare /s/ and /ʃ/ again, pointing to your mouth as you say the sounds so that the children can see the difference in what moves as you say those sounds. Ask the children to repeat /s/ and /ʃ/ and to feel how their mouths move differently for the two sounds.)

Listening and Looking for /ʃ/ at the Beginning of Words

- "Now we're going to listen and look for the /ʃ/ sound in words. Watch my mouth as I say these words. Nod your head yes if /ʃ/ is the first sound in the word I say. Shake your head no if you don't hear /ʃ/ at the beginning of 'the word.'"
- "sheep (*pause*) Yes, I hear the sound /ʃ/ at the beginning of 'sheep.'"
- "shirt (*pause*) Yes, I hear the sound /ʃ/ at the beginning of 'shirt.'"
- "farm (*pause*) No, I don't hear the sound /ʃ/ at the beginning of 'farm.'"
- "shop (*pause*) Yes, I hear /ʃ/ at the beginning of 'shop.'"
- "horse (*pause*) No, I don't hear /ʃ/ at the beginning of 'horse.'"
- "zebra (*pause*) No, I don't hear /ʃ/ at the beginning of 'zebra.'"
- "she (*pause*) Yes, I hear /ʃ/ at the beginning of 'she.'"

Listening and Looking for /ʃ/ in the Beginning, Middle, or End of Words

- "Now all of the words I say are going to have the sound /ʃ/ in the word, but you have to listen very carefully and watch my mouth as I say the words. When I call on someone, your job will be to tell me if you heard the sound /ʃ/ at the beginning (first sound), middle, or end (last sound) of the word. For example, if I say the word 'bush,' the /ʃ/ sound is at the end of the word. 'Bus'—hear the /ʃ/ at the end? If I say 'sheet,' the /ʃ/ sound is the beginning sound in the word."
- shape (beginning)
- mash (end)
- wish (end)
- machine (middle)
- wash (end)
- shine (beginning)
- vacation (middle)
- ocean (middle)
- ship (beginning)
- washing (middle)
- shed (beginning)
- fish (end)

Phoneme /tʃ/ (Digraph *ch*)

Information for the Teacher

- Place: tongue in the middle of mouth (palatal)
- Voicing: quiet (voiceless)
- Manner: affricate (air briefly blocked, then noisy air blowing out)
- Common spellings: *ch*-chair, *tch*-hutch, *ti*-question, *tu*-natural

Information for the Children

- "Today we are talking about the /tʃ/ sound. The letters *ch* make the /tʃ/ sound."
- "The /tʃ/ sound is the sound a choo-choo train makes as it's chugging down the tracks: /tʃ/, /tʃ/, /tʃ/, /tʃ/, /tʃ/, /tʃ/, /tʃ/, /tʃ/." (Move arms like train wheels moving while saying *ch-ch-ch* sounds.)
- "I make the /tʃ/ sound with my tongue in the middle of my mouth, blocking the air and then blowing it out quickly. The /tʃ/ sound is a quiet sound. I just hear air blowing—I don't hear my voice on when I say it."
- "Listen and watch my mouth as I make the /tʃ/ sound: /tʃ/, /tʃ/, /tʃ/, /tʃ/, /tʃ/, /tʃ/."
- "Now you practice saying the /tʃ/ sound several times. Feel where your tongue is in the middle of your mouth. Feel how you block the air and then air blows out just for a little bit. I'll hand out some mirrors to pass around. Look in the mirror as you say /tʃ/ two times, then pass the mirror to the next child."

Listening and Looking for the /tʃ/ Sound by Itself

- "Watch my mouth and listen carefully as I say some sounds. Nod your head yes if you hear and see the /tʃ/ sound. Shake your head no if you don't hear the /tʃ/ sound."
- "/k/ (*pause*) No, that was not the /tʃ/ sound."
- "/tʃ/ (*pause*) Yes, that was the /tʃ/ sound."
- "/dʒ/ (*pause*) That is a hard one. It's not the /tʃ/ sound. We make the /tʃ/ sound somewhat like the /dʒ/ sound, but the /dʒ/ sound is a loud sound. We have our voice on when we say the /tʃ/ sound, but /tʃ/ is a quiet sound with our voice off. Listen again to the difference between /tʃ/ and /tʃ/: /tʃ/ is quiet; the /tʃ/ sound is louder, with our voice on."
- "/w/ (*pause*) No, that was not the /tʃ/ sound."
- "/tʃ/ (*pause*) Yes, that was the /tʃ/ sound."
- "/ʃ/ (*pause*) No, that was not the /tʃ/ sound." (If any children have nodded their heads indicating that it was the /tʃ/ sound, explain that /ʃ/ is a quiet sound that blows air out like the /tʃ/ sound but the /ʃ/ sound is different because air does not get blocked at all when we say /ʃ/ and air gets blown out longer; on the other hand, with the /tʃ/ sound air is blocked and then air is blown out just for a little bit. Compare /tʃ/ and /ʃ/ again. Ask the children to repeat /tʃ/ and /ʃ/ and to feel how their mouths move differently for the two sounds.)
- "/t/ (*pause*) No, that was not the /tʃ/ sound." (If any children have nodded their heads indicat-

ing that it was the /ʧ/ sound, explain that /t/ is a quiet sound like /ʧ/ but the /t/ sound is different because the tongue is right behind the front teeth and /t/ is a little shorter sound. For /ʧ/ the tongue is more in the middle of our mouth and it's a little longer sound. Compare /t/ and /ʧ/ again. Ask the children to repeat /t/ and /ʧ/ and to feel how their tongues move differently for the two sounds.)

- "/ʧ/ (*pause*) Yes, that was the /ʧ/ sound."
- "/s/ (*pause*) No, that was not the /ʧ/ sound."

Listening and Looking for /ʧ/ at the Beginning of Words

- "Now we're going to listen and look for the /ʧ/ sound in words. Watch my mouth as I say these words. Nod your head yes if /ʧ/ is the first sound in the word I say. Shake your head no if you don't hear /ʧ/ at the beginning of 'the word.'"
- "chin (*pause*) Yes, I hear the sound /ʧ/ at the beginning of 'chin.'"
- "chicken (*pause*) Yes, I hear the sound /ʧ/ at the beginning of 'chicken.'"
- "book (*pause*) No, I don't hear the sound /ʧ/ at the beginning of 'book.'"
- "chain (*pause*) Yes, I hear /ʧ/ at the beginning of 'chain.'"
- "shoe (*pause*) No, I don't hear /ʧ/ at the beginning of 'shoe.'"
- "zebra (*pause*) No, I don't hear /ʧ/ at the beginning of 'zebra.'"
- "chair (*pause*) Yes, I hear /ʧ/ at the beginning of 'chair.'"

Listening and Looking for /ʧ/ in the Beginning, Middle, or End of Words

- "Now all of the words I say are going to have the sound /ʧ/ in the word, but you have to listen very carefully and watch my mouth as I say the words. When I call on someone, your job will be to tell me if you heard the sound /ʧ/ at the beginning (first sound), middle, or end (last sound) of the word. For example, if I say the word 'rich,' the /ʧ/ sound is at the end of the word. 'Rich'—hear the /ʧ/ at the end? If I say 'chase,' the /ʧ/ sound is the beginning sound in the word."
- kitchen (middle)
- watch (end)
- chocolate (beginning)
- teacher (middle)
- chick (beginning)
- witch (end)
- pitcher (middle)
- chase (beginning)
- children (beginning)
- match (end)

Phoneme /ŋ/ (Digraph *ng*)

Information for the Teacher

- Place: back of mouth (velar)
- Voicing: voice on (voiced)
- Manner: air passes through the nose (nasal)
- Common spellings: *ng*-song, *n*-think, *nd*-handkerchief
- The /ŋ/ sound only occurs in the medial and final positions of words.

Information for the Children

- "Today we are talking about the /ŋ/ sound. The letters *ng* usually make the /ŋ/ sound.
- "I make the /ŋ/ sound by moving the back part of the tongue up and toward the top of my mouth. When I say the /ŋ/ sound, air comes out of my nose and I can hear my voice."
- "Listen and watch my mouth as I make the /ŋ/ sound: /ŋ/, /ŋ/, /ŋ/, /ŋ/, /ŋ/, /ŋ/, /ŋ/."
- "Now you practice saying the /ŋ/ sound several times. Feel your tongue go way back in your mouth. Feel your voice on in your throat as you say it. I'll hand out some mirrors to pass around. Look in the mirror as you say /ŋ/ two times, then pass the mirror to the next child."

Listening and Looking for the /ŋ/ Sound by Itself

- "Nod your head yes if you hear the /m/ sound. Shake your head no if you don't hear the /m/ sound."
- "/ŋ/ (*pause*) Yes, that was the /ŋ/ sound."
- "/s/ (*pause*) No, that was not the /ŋ/ sound."
- "/k/ (*pause*) No, that was not the /ŋ/ sound."
- "/ŋ/ (*pause*) Yes, that was the /ŋ/ sound."
- "/f/ (*pause*) No, that was not the /ŋ/ sound."
- "/g/ (*pause*) That is a hard one. It's not the /ŋ/ sound. We make the /g/ sound with our tongue near the same place as the /ŋ/ sound, but the /g/ sound is a short sound that comes out of our mouth and the /ŋ/ is a long sound that comes out of our nose. Listen again to the difference between /g/ and /ŋ/. The /g/ sound is short, whereas the /ŋ/ sound is long."
- "/r/ (*pause*) No, that was not the /ŋ/ sound."
- "/ŋ/ (*pause*) Yes, that was the /ŋ/ sound."
- "/n/ (*pause*) No, that was not the /ŋ/ sound." (If any children have nodded their heads indicating that it was the /ŋ/ sound, explain that /n/ is a loud sound that comes out of our nose like the /ŋ/ sound but the /n/ sound is different because the front tip of the tongue goes up behind the front teeth instead of the back of the tongue being near the roof of the mouth for /ŋ/. Compare /n/ and /ŋ/ again, with special attention to feeling the tongue. Ask the children to repeat /n/ and /ŋ/ and to feel how their tongues move differently for the two sounds.)

Listening and Looking for /ŋ/ in the End of Words

- "Now we're going to listen for the /ŋ/ sound in words. Nod your head yes if /ŋ/ is the last sound in the word I say. Shake your head no if you don't hear /ŋ/ at the end of the word."
- "sing (*pause*) Yes, I hear the sound /ŋ/ at the end of 'sing.'"
- "string (*pause*) Yes, I hear the sound /ŋ/ at the end of 'string.'"
- "warm (*pause*) No, I don't hear the sound /ŋ/ at the end of 'warm.'"
- "long (*pause*) Yes, I hear /ŋ/ at end of 'long.'"
- "big (*pause*) No, I don't hear /ŋ/ at the end of 'big.'"
- "slipper (*pause*) No, I don't hear /ŋ/ at the end of 'slipper.'"
- "ring (*pause*) Yes, I hear /ŋ/ at the beginning of 'ring.'"

Listening and Looking for /ŋ/ in the Middle or at the End of Words

- "Now all the words I say are going to have the sound /ŋ/ in the word, but you have to listen very carefully and watch my mouth as I say the words. When I call on you, your job will be to tell me if you heard the sound /ŋ/ in the middle or at the end (last sound) of the word. For example, if I say the word 'song,' the /ŋ/ sound is at the end of the word. 'Song'—hear the /ŋ/ at the end? If I say 'hungry,' the /ŋ/ sound is the middle sound in the word."
- asking (end)
- sharing (end)
- strong (end)
- hanger (middle)
- climbing (end)
- driving (end)
- dancing (end)
- wrong (end)
- singer (middle)

Phonemes /θ/ (*thumb*), /ð/ (*those*) (Digraph *th*)

Information for the Teacher

- Place: tongue between upper and lower teeth (interdental)
- Voicing: quiet (/θ/, voiceless) *or* voice on (/ð/, voiced)
- Manner: fricative (noisy air continuously blowing out)
- Common spellings: *th*-thigh, *th*-the
- The /θ/ and /ð/ sounds are produced without or with the voice, respectively. Because it is difficult for many children to hear the small difference between the voiceless and voiced sounds, it is adviseable to work on the voiceless /θ/ and voiced /ð/ sounds together.

Information for the Children

- "Today we are talking about the /θ/ sound and the /ð/ sound. The letters *th* make either the /θ/ sound or the /ð/ sound."
- "I make the /θ/ or the /ð/ with my tongue touching the bottom of my upper front teeth. My tongue goes in between my two rows of teeth. Sometimes I say /ð/ with my voice on, as in the word 'the.' But I also can say /θ/ without turning on my voice, as in the words 'thing.'"
- "Listen and watch my mouth as I make the /θ/ sound without turning on my voice: /θ/, /θ/, /θ/, /θ/, /θ/, /θ/. Now listen to the sound with my voice on: /ð/, /ð/, /ð/, /ð/, /ð/, /ð/."
- "Now you practice saying the /ð/ sound several times with your voice on. Feel where your tongue goes between your teeth as you say it. Now try to say the /θ/ sound once with your voice on and then the /θ/ once with your voice off. I'll hand out some mirrors to pass around. Look in the mirror as you say /ð/ two times and /θ/ two times, then pass the mirror to the next child."

Listening and Looking for the /θ/ or /ð/ Sound by Itself

- "Watch my mouth and listen carefully as I say some sounds. Nod your head yes if you hear and see the /θ/ or /ð/ sound. Shake your head no if you don't hear the /θ/ or /ð/ sound."
- "/ð/ (*pause*) Yes, that was the /ð/ sound."
- "/r/ (*pause*) No, that was not the /ð/ sound."
- "/m/ (*pause*) No, that was not the /ð/ sound."
- "/θ/ (*pause*) Yes, that was the /θ/ sound."
- "/s/ (*pause*) No, that was not the /ð/ sound."
- "/k/ (*pause*) No, that was not the /ð/ sound."
- "/ð/ (*pause*) Yes, that was the /ð/ sound."
- "/f/ (*pause*) No, that was not the /θ/ sound." (If any children have nodded their heads indicating that it was the /θ/ sound, explain that /f/ is a quiet sound that blows air out like the /θ/ sound but the /f/ sound is different because the top teeth touch the bottom lip whereas the tongue goes between the teeth for /θ/. Compare /f/ and /θ/ again, pointing to your mouth as

you say the sounds so that the children can see the difference in what moves as you say those sounds. Ask the children to repeat /f/ and /θ/ and to feel how their mouths move differently for the two sounds.)

Listening and Looking for /θ/ or /ð/ at the Beginning of Words

- "Now we're going to listen and look for the /θ/ or /ð/ sound in words. Watch my mouth as I say these words. Nod your head yes if /θ/ or /ð/ is the first sound in the word I say. Shake your head no if you don't hear /θ/ or /ð/ at the beginning of the word."
- "thumb (*pause*) Yes, I hear the sound /θ/ at the beginning of 'thumb.'"
- "the (*pause*) Yes, I hear the sound /ð/ at the beginning of 'the.'"
- "shake (*pause*) No, I don't hear the sound /ð/ at the beginning of 'shake.'"
- "they (*pause*) Yes, I hear /ð/ at the beginning of 'they.'"
- "find (*pause*) No, I don't hear /ð/ at the beginning of 'find.'"
- "simple (*pause*) No, I don't hear /ð/ at the beginning of 'simple.'"
- "thing (*pause*) Yes, I hear /θ/ at the beginning of 'thing.'"

Listening and Looking for /θ/ or /ð/ in the Beginning, Middle, or End of Words

- "Now all the words I say are going to have the sound /θ/ or /ð/ in the word, but you have to listen very carefully and watch my mouth as I say the words. When I call on someone, your job will be to tell me if you heard the sound /θ/ or /ð/ at the beginning (first sound), middle, or end (last sound) of the word. For example, if I say the word 'bath,' the /θ/ sound is at the end of the word. 'Bath'—hear the /θ/ at the end? If I say 'thumb,' the /θ/ sound is the beginning sound in the word."
- bother (/ð/, middle)
- smooth (/ð/, end)
- thought (/θ/, beginning)
- together (/ð/, middle)
- these (/ð/, beginning)
- truth (/θ/, end)
- south (/θ/, end)
- author (/θ/, middle)
- thunderstorm (/θ/, beginning)
- nothing (/θ/, middle)
- they (/ð/, beginning)
- soothe (/ð/, end)
- feather (/ð/, middle)

Appendix

Books, Materials, and Alternative Books for Each Class Lesson

This appendix provides titles of the storybooks used in each classroom lesson in Chapter 3 and the materials needed for each lesson. These stories are read aloud by the teacher at each lesson to add appeal to kindergarten children. Many prekindergarten through first-grade storybooks can be used to target various phonemic awareness skills along with enhancing vocabulary, listening skills, and comprehension. Much of the suggested literature accompanying the lessons can be replaced by using another storybook with a similar theme. Examples of alternative literature to use if a suggested book cannot be located are also provided.

The most important aspect to remember as you teach phonemic awareness through literature and activities is to target the skills in a developmental order (e.g., clapping the number of syllables in words [syllable counting] is easier for children than naming the sounds in words [segmenting phonemes]). It is more important to be teaching the appropriate skill than it is to use a specific book. Look at items to target the skill in the suggested book. Adapt to the new book using similar types of questions during the book reading. A list of the suggested book, materials, and alternate books are included here lesson by lesson so the materials can easily be gathered for the whole-class lessons.

Lesson 1
Book
The Itsy Bitsy Spider by Iza Trapani. New York: Scholastic, 1993. ISBN: 0-590-69821-4.

Materials
None needed

Alternative Books
Over in the Meadow by Paul Galdone. New York: Scholastic, 1986. ISBN: 0-590-98044-0.

Lesson 2
Book
It's Raining, It's Pouring by Kin Eagle. Danvers, MA: Whispering Coyote Press, 1994. ISBN: 1-879085-71-2.

Materials

Umbrella (whole-class activity)
Bucket (whole-class and small-group activities)
Box (whole-class and small-group activities)
Pencils (introduction)
Whistle (introduction)
Kazoo/noisemaker (introduction)
Ball (introduction)

Alternative Books

Listen to the Rain by Bill Martin, Jr., & John Archambault. New York: Henry Holt, 1988. ISBN: 0-0805006826.
Rain Rain Rivers by Uri Shulevitz. New York: Farrar, Straus & Giroux. LCN: 73085370/AC.
Peter Spier's Rain by Peter Spier. New York: Doubleday, 1982. ISBN: 0385154844.

Lesson 3

Book

Five Little Ducks by Pamela Paparone. New York: Scholastic, 1995. ISBN: 0-590-96581-6.

Materials

String, rope, or tape to make "duck pond" on floor (whole-class activity)

Alternative Books

Duck in the Truck by Jez Alborough, New York: Scholastic, 2000. ISBN: 0060286857.
Ten Apples Up on Top by Theodore LeSieg. New York: Beginner Books, 1961. ISBN: 0394900197.

Lesson 4

Book

Any Mother Goose rhyme book. A good choice might be: *Hey Diddle Diddle and Other Mother Goose Rhymes*
    by Tomie dePaola. New York: Putnam, 1988. ISBN: 88-11561.

Materials

None needed

Alternative Books

Anna Banana by Joanna Cole. New York: Scholastic, 1989. ISBN: 0688077889.
Hickory, Dickory, Dock by Robin Muller & Suzanne Duranceau. New York: Scholastic, 1992. ISBN:
    059047278X.

Lesson 5

Book

Guess How Much I Love You by Sam McBratney. New York: Scholastic, 1994. ISBN: 0-590-67981-3.

Materials

Four green towels for bushes (whole-class activity)
String/yarn to lay across last circles on rabbit track for finish line (small-group activity)

Alternative Books

I Love You So Much by Carl Norac. New York: Bantam Doubleday Dell, 1988. ISBN: 0385325126.
If You Were My Bunny, by Kate McMullan. New York: Scholastic, 1996. ISBN: 0590527495.

Lesson 6

Book

The Popcorn Shop by Alice Low. New York: Scholastic,, 1993. ISBN: 0-590-4721-X.

Materials

Popcorn (with the book)
Cups to hold popcorn (with the book)
Popcorn for bingo markers (small-group activity)

Alternative Books

Popcorn by Frank Asch. Boston: Houghton Mifflin, 1979. ISBN: 0819310018.

Lesson 7

Book

The Very Hungry Caterpillar by Eric Carle. New York: Philomel, 1987. ISBN: 0-399-20853-4.

Materials

Puppet (whole-class activity)

Alternative Books

Charlie the Caterpillar by Dom De Luise. New York: Simon & Schuster, 1990. ISBN: 0671693581.
I Wish I Were a Butterfly, by James Howe. San Diego: Harcourt Brace Jovanovich, 1987. ISBN: 015200470X.

Lesson 8

Book

There's a Bug in My Mug by Kent Salisbury. New York: McClanahan, 1997. ISBN: 1-56293-931-9.

Materials

Clothing items for introduction choices: socks, shoes, coat, hat, shorts, pants, shirt (introduction)

Alternative Books

The Fish Who Could Wish by John Bush & Korky Paul. Brooklyn, NY: Kane/Miller, 1991. ISBN: 0916291359.
The Caboose Who Got Loose by Bill Peet. Boston: Houghton Mifflin, 1971. ISBN: 0395148057.

Lesson 9

Book

The ABC Mystery by Doug Cushman. New York: HarperCollins, 1993. ISBN: 0-06-021227-6.

Materials

Trench coat, magnifying aglass, hat, for the teacher to dress up as a detective (introduction and whole-class activity)
Three envelopes into which to put three mystery pictures (introduction)
Index cards with one-syllable words written on them of Items in the classroom (whole-class activity)
Prize (stickers or snack, etc.) to find at end of scavenger hunt (whole-class activity)

Alternative Books

Miss Nelson Is Missing by Harry Allard. Boston: Houghton Mifflin, 1977. ISBN: 0395252962.
Herbie Hamster, Where Are You by Terence Blacker. New York: Random House, 1990. ISBN: 0679808388.

Lesson 10

Each child needs a pencil or some other writing instrument.

Lesson 11

Book

What Am I?: An Animal Guessing Game by Iza Trapani. Boston: Whispering Coyote Press, 1992. ISBN: 1-879085-66-6.

Materials

Ball (whole-class activity)
Tape (whole-class activity)
Chips or tokens for Bingo (small-group activity)

Alternative Books

Says Who?: A Pop-up Book of Animal Sounds by David A. Carter. New York: Simon & Schuster, 1993. ISBN: 0671729233.
Baby Animals by Margaret Wise Brown. New York: Random House, 1989. ISBN: 0394820401.

Lesson 12

Book

Kids Celebrate the Alphabet by Teresa Walsh. Everett, WA: Warren. ISBN 1-57029-162-4.

Materials

Puppet (introduction)
Bag (small-group activity)
Objects to put in bag (pencil, pen, paper, rock, ring, something red, dime, duck, doll, tape, tack, toy) (small-group activity)

Alternative Books

Anno's Alphabet: An Adventure in Imagination by Mitsumasa Anno. New York: Crowell, 1974. ISBN: 0690005407.

The Letters are Lost by Lisa Campbell Ernst. New York: Scholastic, 1996. ISBN: 067086336X.

Lesson 13

Book

The Caboose Who Got Loose by Bill Peet. Boston: Houghton-Mifflin, 1971. ISBN: 0-395-14805-7.

Materials

None needed

Alternative Books

Thomas Gets Tricked by Rev. W. Awdry. New York: Random House, 1989. ISBN: 0679801086.

Little Red Caboose by Steve Metzger. New York: Scholastic, 1999. ISBN: 0590635980.

The Little Engine That Could by Watty Piper. New York: Scholastic, 1976. ISBN: 0448400413.

Lesson 14

Book

The Icky Sticky Anteater by Dawn Bentley. Santa Monica, CA: Piggy Toes Press, 2000. ISBN: 1-58117-121-8.

Materials

Sticky tack (whole-class activity)

Alternative Books

The Very Quiet Cricket by Eric Carle. New York: Philomel Books, 1990. ISBN: 0399218858.

The Grouchy Ladybug by Eric Carle. New York: Harper, 1977. ISBN: 0690013922.

Lesson 15

Book

If You Give a Mouse a Cookie by Laura Joffe Numeroff. New York: HarperCollins, 1985. ISBN: 0-06-024586-7.

Materials

Oreo cookie (introduction)

"Hot Potato" game or some similar object to pass around (whole-class activity)

Music to play (whole-class activity)

Alternative Books

Mmm, Cookies! by Robert Munsch. New York: Scholastic, 2000. ISBN: 059089032.

The Mouse and the Potato by Thomas Berger. Edinburgh: Floris Books, 1990. ISBN: 0863151035.

Lesson 16

Book

Jump Frog Jump by Robert Kalan. New York: Greenwillow Books, 1981. ISBN: 0-688-13954-X.

Materials

Green towels/pretend lily pads (whole-class activity)
Tongue blades/popsicle sticks (small-group activity)
Puppet (introduction)

Alternative Books

In the Small, Small Pond by Denise Fleming. New York: Scholastic, 1993. ISBN: 0805022643.
It's Mine by Leo Lionni. New York: Scholastic, 1986. ISBN: 039487000X.
Froggy Goes to School by Jonathon London. New York: Scholastic, 1996. ISBN: 0670867268.

Lesson 17

Book

One Fish, Two Fish, Red Fish, Blue Fish by Dr. Suess. New York: Random House, 1988. ISBN: 0-394-90013-8.

Materials

A small swimming pool or pretend pond (large blue piece of paper) (whole-class activity)
Fishing pole with a magnet (whole-class activity)
Bag, net, or container to hold fish (whole-class activity)
Paper clips (whole-class activity)

Alternative Books

Fish Is Fish by Leo Lionni. New York: Scholastic, 1970. ISBN: 0394904400.
The Rainbow Fish by Marcus Pfister. New York: North-South Books, 1992. ISBN: 1558580107.

Lesson 18

Book

Franklin in the Dark by Paulette Bourgeois and Brenda Clark. New York: Scholastic, 1986. ISBN: 0-590-44506-5

Materials

Flashlight (introduction)
Sheet (whole-class activity)
Small box (whole-class activity)

Alternative Books

Is It Dark? Is It Light? by Mary D. Lankford. New York: Scholastic, 1991. ISBN: 0679815791.
A Dark Dark Tale by Ruth Brown. New York: Dial, 1981. ISBN: 0803700938.

Lesson 19

Book

Big Sarah's Little Boots by Paulette Bourgeois & Brenda Clark. New York: Scholastic, 1987. ISBN: 0-590-42623-0.

Materials

Scissors (introduction)
Dolls or stuffed animals (five) (whole-class activity)
Five small chairs (whole-class activity)
Unifix cubes for small-group activity (small-group activity)

Alternative Books

Boots by Anne Schreiber. New York: Scholastic, 1994. ISBN: 059027371X.
Jesse Bear, What Will You Wear? by Nancy White Carlstrom. New York: Macmillan, 1986. ISBN: 002717350X.

Lesson 20

Book

It Begins with an A by Stephanie Calmenson. New York: Scholastic, 1993. ISBN: 0-590-48173-8.

Materials

Plastic eggs that open

Alternative Books

Q is for Duck by Mery Elting & Michael Folsom. New York: Houghton Mifflin/Clarion Books, 1980. ISBN: 0395294371.
Albert B. Cub and Zebra: An Alphabet Storybook by Mirra Ginsburg. New York: Penguin, 1977. ISBN: 0690013507.

Index